AF450105

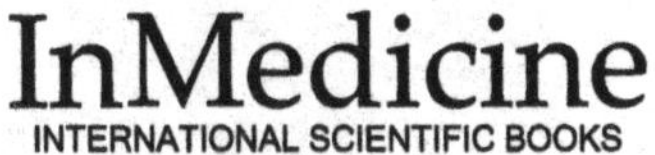

InMedicine
INTERNATIONAL SCIENTIFIC BOOKS

una collana a cura di
Pasquale Bacco

Nutrition and sport with diabetes
di Eleonora Campagnoli
prima edizione: 2025
© 2025, Santelli Editore

Santelli Editore
Via F. Filzi, 3
Cinisello B. - Milano - 20092
340.9481047

Santelli Editore è un marchio di proprietà del Gruppo Editoriale Santelli.
www.grupposantelli.it

ELEONORA CAMPAGNOLI

NUTRITION AND SPORT WITH DIABETES

In the shoes of an athlete

S

INDEX

DEDICATION

Welcome to my journey through life with diabetes! I'm excited to share my story with you, and I have three main goals in mind:

Giving you a glimpse into my life with diabetes: I want to take you on a journey through my daily experiences, sharing my unique perspective and the data that has shaped my path. This book is for anyone who wants to understand the challenges, triumphs, and strategies I've learned as a diabetic athlete. I hope to inspire and guide you on your own diabetes journey!

Helping you tackle diabetes challenges: By sharing my story, I aim to deepen your understanding of the intricacies of diabetes. It's a 24/7 job that can be mentally and physically draining. But I've learned some valuable tools to manage hyperglycemia and glucose instability, and I'm excited to share them with you!

The power of mindset: Living with diabetes can be a rollercoaster of emotions, but I've learned that it's essential to stay balanced. I've come to realize that "don't let the highs get too high, or the lows get too low" is more than just a phrase - it's a way of life. Finding mental and physical stability has been key to achieving my goals, and I hope to inspire you to do the same with my story making you feel like you are in my shoes!

Encourage Health Care Professional Consultation: The information provided in this book is based on personal experiences, research, and insights from living with Type 1 diabetes and participating in sports. It is intended for informational and inspirational purposes only and should not be considered medical or professional advice.

Readers are encouraged to consult with qualified healthcare professionals, including physicians, nutritionists, and fitness experts, before making any changes to their medical treatments.

1. INTRODUCTION

Welcome to my story, with the aim to make you feel what it means to be in My Shoes as a sports woman, living abroad, with diabetes! I am Eleonora, born in 1995 in Turin, Italy. Turin is a beautiful city in northern Italy, nestled at the base of the Alps. The city has always been a source of inspiration for me, filled with art exhibitions, music festivals, and science conferences that sparked my scientific passion. Growing up in Turin, I learned to appreciate the balance of life's highs and lows, a principle I now carry forward: Never Too High, Never Too Low. The same principle I carry forward in my diabetes life, where I look for a fine balance between pushing myself to the limit and giving myself enough time to rest and recover, avoiding blood glucose highs and lows roller coaster.

During my teenage years, I graduated with a degree in Molecular Biotechnology from the University of Turin. While at university, a professor recognized my courage and readiness for change, and this encouraged me to broaden my horizons. This led me to leave my beloved Italy and family to pursue a master's degree in oncology at the Vrije University of Amsterdam. My passion for science has always been strong. Fascinated by the biological processes of the human body, I am constantly questioning how to influence them to improve human well-being. By embracing the mantra of Never Too High, Never Too Low, I navigated these transitions with resilience and curiosity.

During my time in the Netherlands, I worked in cancer hospitals and pharmaceutical companies such as Johnson & Johnson. Currently, I am a consultant engineer in Digital Manufacturing and Quality System Validation at Capgemini Engineering. During these years I have grown into the role of Project Coordinator, Business Analyst and Scrum Master. However, work is not everything to me. In my free time, I volunteer as a Swim Director and Nutrition associate for the Amsterdam Triathlon and Cycling Club. These roles allowed me to channel my passion for sports into the club and train as part of a team to complete my sporting challenges with diabetes. It's in these moments of teamwork and personal challenge that I remind myself to maintain a balance, staying Never Too High, Never Too Low.

Despite my busy schedule, I find time to read triathlon books and take courses in Sport Performance and Nutrition. Finally, I am proud to share my Nutrition and Life Coach certificates. Although my life might seem very serious, I am passionate about savoring life's small moments, enjoying its beauty, and being grateful for every breath. I deeply believe in the power of change and challenges, both in life and sports. I have tried my hand at various activities, including tennis, boxing, spinning, climbing, biking, swimming, and running. This varied approach helps me keep perspective, embracing the Never Too High, Never Too Low philosophy in all aspects of my life.

Most importantly, I have lived with Type 1 diabetes since I was three years old. I cannot remember life without it, but I have turned diabetes into a strength—a unique part of me that sets me apart. Unfortunately, autoimmune diseases, like diabetes, often come in pairs. Since 2013 I have been suffering from Hashimoto hypothyroidism, which strongly affects my metabolism.

Currently, my focus is on preparing for triathlons. I have completed sprint and olympic distances triathlons as of June 2022. I was proud to complete the Amsterdam Half Marathon in 2023, along with the Ironman 70.3 in Cervia, Italy. These challenges motivate me to invest in myself, study, and improve my diabetes management.

When I decided to call this book "In the shoes of an athlete" I wanted to convey more than just my journey with Type 1 diabetes. I wanted to invite you to step into my world and see life from my perspective—not to gain sympathy, but to share an experience. Living with diabetes has shaped the way I approach everything: from everyday decisions to the intense demands of athletic training and competition. But this book isn't just about me. It's about the mindset and determination needed to overcome the hurdles that life throws at us, whether it's a chronic illness, a personal challenge, or a goal that seems out of reach.

"Nutrition and Sport with Diabetes" is an invitation. It's a chance for you to walk alongside me, to see the obstacles and triumphs through my eyes, and perhaps to reflect on your own journey. Whether you're living with diabetes or facing different challenges, I believe that the steps I've taken can resonate with anyone who's had to navigate their own unique path.

In these pages, you'll find the raw realities of my life with diabetes, but also the strategies and mindset that have helped me thrive. I want this book to empower you, to show you that no matter what shoes you're walking in, you have the strength to keep going, one step at a time.

2. LIFE CHAPTERS

This book is for everyone, whether you're managing diabetes or simply looking for inspiration. I'm excited to share this journey with you, and I hope you'll find strength, insight, and hope in these pages. Let's walk in my shoes, this path together, starting from my life chapters.

One day, my mom asked me to give a title to the different chapters of my life. In that moment, I could clearly picture four distinct stories that characterize me.

THE RUN

In 1999, when I was just three years old, my life took a sudden and unexpected turn. I was diagnosed with type 1 diabetes, a condition that would become a constant companion in my journey. I vividly remember being at home, enjoying the innocence of childhood, when everything changed. In an instant, I found myself on my mother's shoulder, running down a long, white corridor towards a bright light. I was holding something in my hand—a long line that I always imagined was the string of a balloon. It was an IV line connected to my arm, a tether to the medical world that would help manage my new condition. A nurse was running beside us, pushing the IV stand, her presence a blur of urgency and care.

This was my first lesson in the importance of balance as I started to experience the peaks and difficulties of living with diabetes. As the days in the hospital passed, they left only faint impressions in my memory. However, one moment stands out clearly, marked by both hunger and joy.

I remember feeling an insatiable hunger, a sensation that seemed to consume my tiny frame. The nurses were firm in their refusal to give me food, adhering to the strict protocols necessary for my treatment. After what felt like endless complaining, I was finally granted half a banana. It was the best half-banana of my life, a small victory in a world suddenly dominated by medical restrictions. In that moment, the concept of never too high, never too low was embodied in the simplest of acts—finding immense satisfaction in a small portion, understanding the need for moderation and patience.

Amidst the sterile hospital environment, one evening brought a wave of unexpected delight. My uncle Andrea came to visit, carrying a gift that would become a treasured memory. It was a Barbie doll, not just any Barbie, but one engaged in gymnastics, possibly rowing on a tiny rowing machine. To my three-year-old self, it was a beacon of joy and normalcy in a sea of medical procedures and unfamiliar faces. The Barbie even made sounds, causing me to laugh uncontrollably. Despite the expectation to maintain silence in the dark hospital room, my laughter broke the rules, filling the space with light and happiness. This joyful rebellion was a perfect example of living Never Too High, Never Too Low, embracing moments of unrestrained joy even in challenging circumstances.

Looking back, that hospital stay was the beginning of a lifelong journey of balancing the ups and downs of living with diabetes. The

IV line, the half-banana, and the laughing Barbie were more than just memories—they were lessons in maintaining equilibrium. As I grew, this principle of balance became integral to my approach to life, guiding me through the myriad of challenges and triumphs that lay ahead.

TEARS FOR INDEPENDENCE

"Sur le pont d'Avignon, l'on y danse, l'on y danse, Sur le pont d'Avignon, l'on y danse tous en rond." On the bus headed to Avignon for a middle school trip, we were singing this popular French song. I was by the window, sitting next to my best friend. All the parents were looking up at us, waving their hands and sending kisses, some of them almost crying.

The French teacher took the bus microphone and began reminding us about the beautiful week ahead. The most important part was that we were free from our parents! Everyone on the bus started shouting with joy and clapping their hands. Everyone except for me. My mom was on the bus, coming along to support the teachers in managing my diabetes for the full trip.

At that time, I was fully independent in measuring my glucose and injecting insulin, making my own decisions about the carbohydrates amounts. On that bus, I turned towards the window and let a couple of tears fall from my eyes. Tears for independence. I remember thinking how foolish I was; I should be happy my mom was there for me! She did it for me, right? Later, I understood she also did it for herself, for my father, for the teachers, and for me.

I also came to realize that being a parent is one of the hardest things in life, with no right or wrong. I immensely thank my mother for dedicating her life and partly sacrificing her career to take care of me as a child with diabetes. This moment marked the beginning of my journey towards seeking freedom, trust, and independence.

CAN'T STOP EATING

When my grandparents passed away, it felt like a significant part of my life crumbled. Before that moment, I was seeing them every day, I was spending every summer and winter holiday with them. They were a solid brick in the foundation of my life, and their loss felt like an earthquake that destroyed my family, creating a chain of events that left us shattered.

After such a tragedy, you must deal with the consequences. Our familial "house" was destroyed, and we needed to work together to rebuild it or compromise to find a new one—perhaps less perfect, but different. Many mistakes were made, many wounds were opened, and eventually, the four of us found separate, different homes, different cities. Although still a family.

During two years of suffering, I searched for support and answers. I asked myself how I can stop my compulsive eating behavior or how I can find myself again regaining the joy of life.

Diabetes had become overwhelming, leading to an eating disorder that severely impacted my mental health and diabetes management. Unfortunately, I did not find the support I needed from my family; this period became a significant learning moment for me. At some point, something in my mind switched. I found my own answers, developed strategies, and discovered the willpower to change my life.

ROLLING HILLS

In Amsterdam, I found friends, love, and a house along with a stable job. It was there that I discovered my passions: triathlon, nutrition and helping others. Today, my life is a mix of ups and downs, a sea of stability interspersed with a storm of challenges—much like biking on rolling hills. Now, I can pause and reflect on the many steep hills I have already climbed with My Shoes. Together, we can enjoy the view of the beautiful ones ahead, with a clear blue sky above.

3. THE HISTORY

Type 1 diabetes (T1D) is a chronic autoimmune condition in which the body's immune system mistakenly attacks and destroys insulin-producing beta cells in the pancreas. This leads to a lifelong dependency on exogenous insulin to regulate blood glucose levels. The global burden of T1D is significant, affecting millions of individuals across all age groups, though it is most commonly diagnosed in children and young adults.

The prevalence of T1D is increasing worldwide, with an estimated 1.1 million children and adolescents living with the disease as of 2023. However, the total number of people with T1D, including adults, is much higher.

The turning point in the history of T1D came in 1921 when Canadian researchers Frederick Banting and Charles Best, along with J.J.R. Macleod and James Collip discovered insulin. This breakthrough transformed T1D from a fatal disease to a manageable condition.

Before the insulin discovery, the most common treatment involved severely restricting carbohydrate intake and overall caloric consumption to reduce blood sugar levels. Diabetic patients were forced to follow this restricting diet while hospitalized but incapable to keep this eating behavior during their daily life, resulting in being hospitalized again shortly.

An article subtitled "An Analysis of Failure" was published in 1973 and reported the survey results of diabetic patients. Diabetologists, along with their physician colleagues, concluded that their patients were either unwilling or incapable of following the dietary advice they were given. They believed that a diet restricting what patients could eat was not worth whatever benefits might be experienced in the future. They felt that the immediate burden of the disease was not equal to the burden of dietary restriction. Therefore, injecting as much insulin as the patients needed to keep going with their lifestyle was the simple's solution.

Years later, in 2009, as suggested by Dr. Sawyer and Dr. Gale, physicians treating diabetic patients assumed that their patients would prefer to take whatever drugs necessary to control their blood sugar rather than adhere to a diet.

I believe that understanding the history of how this troublesome situation developed is important for critically thinking our way out and taking the next steps for improvement. Even today, following a diet is challenging for most of us. For myself, suffering from Diabetes T1 and Hashimoto Hypothyroidism, I strongly believe that restricting carbohydrates is the way forward, in a society where carbohydrate intake is abused.

I do not demonize carbohydrates, but I would say I restrict them during the day where I am not training. I allow myself to eat them in a "smart" way. What does it mean? I am planning my meal to reach carbohydrates only if they are about to be burned, without creating an increased insulin demand.

In my opinion, taking whatever drug necessary, in this case injecting as much insulin needed to eat whatever, feels wrong to myself.

A combination of sport and careful nutrition is essential to minimize the use of insulin. Insulin should help to assist in diabetes management and not be used as the key element to get our glucose values on target, without paying good attention to diet and exercise.

In Italy, before the purification of insulin in the 19th century, the animal diet was advocated by Doctor Arnoldo Cantani of the University of Pavia. Doctor Cantani was certain that the principal cause of diabetes was the excessive consumption of sugar and starch. He stated that "the remedy of diabetes is not in the drugstore but in the kitchen," a sentiment with which many diabetologists would still agree. Cantani prescribed a diet of only meat and fat, followed with absolute rigor and complete perseverance.

The "Cantani" approach is the foundation of what I have metabolized and elaborated for myself. Nutrition is the real remedy for living with diabetes minimizing the long-term consequences. Shaping my eating habits towards more vegetables and proteins has changed my life, not only making me feel less sleepy after the meal, less tired in the morning and without craving sugar after dinner but also taught me rigor and discipline.

Only in the early twentieth century did diabetologists develop their thinking on how to best treat the disease, with the discovery of insulin itself. All they knew was that those diagnosed with diabetes had elevated sugar in their blood or urine, and they made lowering these numbers the focus of their therapies.

With the discovery of insulin, what was previously recommended for diabetes patients, such as a diet low in carbohydrates, became obsolete. Free eating became the new way of treating the disease, shifting the focus to the right amount of insulin to be injected. This shift in mindset, induced by the difficulties patients had in following a diet and the discovery of insulin allowing them to eat liberally, still nowadays lacks proof that it is the best way to treat the disease.

I had a brief discussion with a couple of diabetologists and I asked them if we know the real consequences of high insulin doses over time on the human body. The answer was "We cannot say exactly". I kept going with a follow up question. My wonder was if it is better to have the glucose in range all the time by injecting high amounts of insulin or is it better to have the glucose level slightly higher with less insulin in the blood? The answer was that we don't know. Currently we do not know if this synthetic insulin will have side effects on a long term on other areas of the body.

Several individuals, including myself, have tried a low-carb diet to reduce the insulin response. I strongly support the idea that a diet should be personalized as each individual has a different body and metabolism, but speaking from my experience, as a female suffering from type 1 diabetes and hypothyroidism, I can attest to several benefits of following it, or at least restrict the amount of carbohydrates during days lacking of physical activity.

I would like to clarify that when I refer to a "low-carb diet," I mean reducing the intake of carbohydrates to below 130 grams per day, but not eliminating them completely. The benefits I have noticed include weight loss, reduced HbA1c levels over time (12-24 months), and lower blood fats such as triglycerides and cholesterol. A lower amount of carbohydrates has improved my quality of life, limited my exogenous insulin requirements, improved my glucose stability, and resulted in stable flat lines on my CGM. I did not notice any increased risk of hypoglycemia or ketoacidosis.

As Gary Taubes suggests in his book "Rethinking Diabetes," it is quite possible that a carbohydrate-rich diet for patients with diabetes, no matter how well covered by insulin therapy, could cause harm compared to a diet low in carbohydrates. In type 1 diabetes, the carbohydrate-rich diet, and the insulin necessary to cover those carbohydrates may be responsible for both long-term complications and short-term issues—the hyperglycemic swings and hypoglycemic reactions that make the disease so difficult to live with. Although the evidence from base medicine fails us here, the evidence supporting the standard care is weak, and diabetologists have never properly tested it against anything else.

From here, I would like to step in with my experience and data analysis, proposing a new mindful method of eating within a healthy lifestyle. The low-carbohydrate diet does not mean the absence of carbohydrates, but rather eating them in a mindful way. By planning our meals to avoid unnecessary insulin doses and focusing on reducing glucose spikes and, therefore, the insulin response, we can create a shift in perspective that is necessary if current approaches to managing diabetes are indeed inappropriate.

4. MY METHOD

The traditional, so-called conventional, approach to diabetes management focuses on maintaining stable blood glucose levels through regular monitoring, standard insulin therapy, a balanced diet with careful carbohydrate counting, and general exercise recommendations.

In contrast, my approach takes diabetes management to a more personalized level, especially for those who lead active lifestyles. I emphasize the importance of incorporating regular daily exercise, with a well-structured plan that balances both strength training and cardio. This routine not only improves overall fitness but also enhances insulin sensitivity and helps maintain better glucose control.

My personal approach to nutrition, shaped by my body type involves a low-carb diet, with careful timing of carbohydrate intake around physical activity— before and/or after exercise—to provide the necessary energy while keeping blood sugar levels stable. This strategy is complemented by personalized insulin adjustments that consider the daily variations in physical activity and individual metabolic responses.

Furthermore, I place a strong emphasis on developing a positive and resilient mindset. Living with diabetes and pursuing an active lifestyle requires mental strength, and my approach includes strategies to cultivate this resilience, ensuring that individuals can overcome challenges and remain motivated.

Overall, my method integrates regular exercise, tailored nutrition, personalized insulin management, and mental resilience to empower individuals with diabetes to live active, healthy, and fulfilling lives.

MY DIABETES HACKS

The conventional wisdom in diabetes management suggests that with the proper administration of insulin, individuals with diabetes can eat whatever they want, whenever they want. While this statement is technically accurate, it overlooks the broader picture of what is truly necessary for optimal health and long-term diabetes management. Insulin is a crucial tool, but it is not the only factor that allows us to lead a balanced life. My approach emphasizes that effective diabetes management involves more than just insulin—it requires a holistic strategy that integrates nutrition, regular physical activity, and stress management.

My belief is rooted in science and personal experience: a balanced, low-carbohydrate diet, combined with consistent daily exercise, promotes greater glucose stability, and reduces the need for large doses of insulin. Insulin itself is not the "bad guy," but the body's insulin response can be problematic if it leads to excessive glucose fluctuations and higher insulin requirements over time. Research has shown that minimizing insulin response over the long term can contribute to better overall health, reducing the risk of complications associated with diabetes.

The method I advocate for reducing insulin response involves a careful combination of balanced nutrition and daily physical activity. By adopting a low-carb diet and engaging in regular exercise, I've noticed significant improvements in glucose stability, a reduced need for insulin, and better overall metabolic health.

BENEFITS OF REDUCING INSULIN RESPONSE

My personal experience made me conclude that the benefits of reducing insulin response are several, such as increased glucose stability, reduction in fat mass and body weight, and decreased body inflammation.

In my experience, I gradually increased my physical activity and this led me to lowering insulin doses. It leads to more stable blood glucose levels, reducing the risk of both hyperglycemia and hypoglycemia therefore an enhanced glucose stability.

A balanced diet and a healthy exercise routine, helped me to reduce insulin doses and create less glucose variability. Over time, I noticed that less insulin in the system helped me decrease fat mass, making it easier to maintain a healthy body weight.

Many doctors recognised a huge inflammation in my body, every time I had an appointment. What I noticed, after implementing a balanced diet with a restricted amount of carbohydrates during the days where less physical activity was involved was an enhanced glucose stability. This led me to decrease my insulin doses and overtime helped me reduce fat mass. Fat mass is associated with lower levels of chronic inflammation, which is beneficial for overall health.

REDUCING GLUCOSE SPIKES

One of my main goals is to reduce the glucose fluctuations. If the glucose increases sharply and fast it can be considered a glucose spike. When blood sugar spikes after eating, it can leave you feeling tired, lethargic and moody. Over time, chronic blood sugar issues can put you at risk for conditions like kidney disease, heart disease and even dementia. Following are my strategies to decrease the chances of glucose spikes, that I adopt every day.

- Savoury Breakfast: Starting the day with a low-carb, high-protein breakfast helps prevent early glucose spikes.
- Post-Meal Activity: A 10-minute walk after every meal can significantly improve glucose uptake and prevent spikes.
- Avoid Snacking: Reducing the frequency of meals helps control insulin levels and reduces the likelihood of glucose fluctuations.
- Balanced Meals: Combining carbohydrates with proteins and healthy fats slows down glucose absorption and moderates' insulin response.

This approach empowered me to achieve better control over my condition by focusing on lifestyle factors that enhance insulin sensitivity and minimize the need for large insulin doses. It represents a shift from traditional diabetes management towards a more proactive and holistic strategy that prioritizes long-term health and well-being.

If you like, have a look at the hacks I use to better manage diabetes. These hacks aim to be a source of inspiration and motivation. Diabetes is a 24 hour job without weekends and holidays but sharing the knowledge and the successful strategies can help others to improve their conditions. Motivation goes up and down and it is difficult to push through some hard days. It is very easy to slip and stop following the nutrition guidelines and the training plan. Even when I follow all the right "steps", I need to face hyperglycemia events. They are particularly frustrating but I found a way to handle all of these situations with some simple hacks.

My deepest wish is to be a guide and push anyone in need to take a step forward towards your goals.

HYPERGLYCEMIA HACKS

- Increase gradually the insulin doses (always ask for medical advice).
- Wait at least 2-3 hours before correcting again with additional insulin (always ask for medical advice).
- Avoid sweets and processed food.
- Move extra 15 minutes every day.

Stay positive, treat yourself with something nice. If you are training, always keep the focus on the performance side, instead of focusing on insulin and glucose levels.

MOTIVATION HACKS

- Stay positive, enjoy the journey.
- Treat yourself with something you love once a week! For me it is a nice massage.
- Focus on improving performance.
- Write down your goal in a SMART way.

TRAINING HACKS

- Structured plan.
- One or two cardio sessions.
- One or two strength sessions.
- One session yoga or meditation.

DATE	7:00-8:00	12:00-13:00	18:00-19:00	19:00-20:00
MON	STRENGHT			EASY BIKE
TUE		LONG RUN		SWIM
WED			STRENGHT	INTERVAL RUN
THU	STRENGHT			INTERVAL BIKE
FRI	SWIM	YOGA		
SAT		LONG BIKE		
SUN		LONG SWIM		YOGA

The table serves as a structured example for a training week.

NUTRITION HACKS

- Structured plan.
- Calculate the amount of Kcal you need (always ask for medical advice).
- Calculate the amount of protein you need.
- Calculate the amount of carbohydrates in every meal.

5. MILESTONES

On June 19th, 2022, I completed my first triathlon! This was a monumental achievement for me and my life with diabetes. After crossing the finish line, a few tears fell, followed by a cascade of thoughts.

Doctors always say you can have a normal life with diabetes, but no one tells you about the thousand different feelings you will experience over the years. "Why me?!" "Enough!" "I am so happy I have diabetes because I get free chocolate when I am low." The reality of diabetes is that with every injection, you face both physical and psychological pain. You have to breathe deeply through the burning sensation under your skin for several minutes, often dealing with immediate bleeding and long-term black spots on your legs and arms. "Is the injection painful?" "No, it's okay."

No one tells you that the more you eat, the more insulin you need, and the greater the sense of hunger you will feel. No one mentions the significant psychological impact of this disease, amplified by the lack of a cure. In daily life, injecting insulin is not just inconvenient; it is scary, painful, and attracts stares. Travelling light and spontaneous is impossible. You have to carry a massive set of supplies everywhere, with replacements for every pen, needle, scanner, and sensor, ready for any possible incident.

No one tells you that to practice sports, you have to plan hours in advance, work twice as hard, and put in double the effort to achieve the same results as your friends. It takes days and years of practice to perform two or three hours of physical activity, calculating what to eat, when, and how.

No one tells you that you won't sleep well anymore, waking up multiple times to drink water, eat sugar, and measure glucose levels. No one tells you that you will gain weight more easily, be more prone to muscle inflammation, and experience slower muscle recovery. They tell you to live a normal life, and luckily, in the end, you will. However, they don't mention the immense sacrifice and commitment required to make it possible.

Turn your weakness into your strength!

AMBASSADOR FOR FID

Two years later, in March 2024, I participated as an Ambassador for the Italian Diabetes Foundation at the "Advanced Technology and Diabetes Treatment" (ATTD) congress in Florence. This was another significant milestone in my journey, a path marked by changes, failures, and achievements that brought me to this point. My presence at the congress was not only a chance to network and meet people from different pharmaceutical industries, to which sometimes I collaborate, and doctors from all over Europe, but also to embrace the vibrant energy of the event with all the new innovations about diabetes technology.

New advanced technologies are emerging to help manage diabetes: better continuous glucose monitors (CGMs), insulin pumps combining insulin and glucagon, and predictive algorithms. I was really impressed thinking about how much progress had been made since 1999, when I was diagnosed with diabetes T1. However, technology is not everything and it will not solve all the diabetes management problems, at least for now.

My most important diabetes lesson I learned the hard way myself, is to always rely on feelings before blindly following the data, as technology can still fail.

ATTD showcased promising treatments, with hopes for broader application in the future. My conference's takeaway was that a healthy lifestyle characterized by a structured exercise plan and personalized nutrition is what makes the difference together with innovation in diabetes care. I had time to reflect on the profound impact of diabetes, mental and physical, reminding myself of the urgency to put my health first in order to arrive healthy in the future.

Anything can be achieved with a positive and determined mindset. I strongly believe that the successful adoption and maintenance of comprehensive behavioral changes in our lifestyle improves glycemic control. This belief is something I have tried and demonstrated as a diabetic patient and athlete.

This bumpy road involves identifying the root causes of harmful behaviors and addressing the reasons behind them—why, where, when, and what. The real benefit of this process is the creation of a new, powerful inner motivation that will enable you to achieve your goals.

6. MY MISSION

Diabetes will be the health challenge of the next millennium. According to the latest data from the International Diabetes Federation (IDF) more than half a billion people live with diabetes worldwide. In Italy it is estimated that almost five million people suffer from this disease. One million of them are people who do not know that they suffer from diabetes, about 4 million are at risk of developing it and 496 people die every year from it.

Improving the lifestyle of people with diabetes is the real challenge, alleviating the everyday burden. Data shows how physical activity contributes to weight loss, makes muscles consume glucose and therefore lower blood glucose, increasing insulin sensitivity, correcting one possible cause of diabetes. Physical activity increases HDL cholesterol (the good one) and reduces blood pressure, improving many risk factors for chronic complications.

This diary explains my journey in optimizing my diabetes management through nutrition, exercise, body changes, and developing my own method to achieve results. First, I became aware of my body and how it reacts to different foods and sports. I identified the problems, created a foundation for change, implemented small adjustments, and kept track of my progress while embracing both failures and successes. This journey has led me to where I am today, with significant achievements and a strong desire to share my knowledge.

My goal is to shift the current mentality, which often focuses solely on glucose values and insulin doses, towards a healthier lifestyle. I advocate for the implementation of cognitive behavioral therapies alongside medical treatments. By doing so, we can achieve better overall health and well-being for those living with diabetes.

PROBLEM IDENTIFICATION

I consider myself a very active person, needing to channel my energy into my passion, sport. When I train, I start smiling, transporting myself to a happy and peaceful place where nothing else matters. When I started writing this book, it was during spring 2022, it was meant to be a personal diary, to deep dive into my diabetes management. At the time, I was training a lot, feeling like my nutrition was good enough but I was not managing to lose weight and build muscles. The glucose was inside the range parameters but still fluctuating a lot between hypoglycemia and hyperglycemia. Lastly, my body was constantly inflamed and tired.

Throughout my experience with diabetes, it has been a journey filled with frustration and desire to better understand the condition. Over the past 20 years, there have been times when I felt like there was a missing piece of the puzzle. I have come across doctors who, despite their expertise, struggled to fully grasp the complex relationship between my diabetes, nutrition, and exercise. Nutritionists have been helpful but often lacked insight into how sports impact diabetes, and personal trainers excelled in fitness but lacked knowledge about diabetes. This search for a holistic approach ignited a passion within me.

I aim to be a mentor for others, providing the support and understanding that I lacked. This is important to me because I have personally experienced the feeling of isolation that comes from being misunderstood by those who are supposed to help us.

My goal is to fill in these gaps in knowledge using my unique skills and experiences. The main difference in my approach is that insulin alone is not the only solution for managing diabetes. To reach optimal HbA1c levels, there are other things we can also do. I have discovered research showing that avoiding spikes in glucose levels is crucial for managing diabetes through a low carb diet. This can reduce the need for insulin, improve HbA1c levels, and help with weight loss over time. My strategy for reducing insulin response involves a combination of a balanced low carb diet, smart nutrition choices, and daily physical activity.

STRATEGY DISCOVERY

Living with type 1 diabetes means that the relationship between insulin and glucose in my body is very important. I love sports, which help me stay active and healthy. Being active not only helps me control my blood sugar levels and reduce my insulin intake, but it also has a positive effect on my mental well-being. However, life sometimes gets in the way, with family responsibilities, work, illness, or other obligations. For me, it's all about setting priorities and making sure to always keep my health in mind. Staying active is crucial for managing my diabetes but also my mental health. I can see a noticeable difference in my daily or weekly blood sugar levels when I have been active compared to when I have not been as active. Through observation and data collection I have noticed how living an active lifestyle positively impacts how I manage my diabetes.

My goal was identified, the optimization of my diabetes management through sport and nutrition. To reach this goal I knew I would have paid a high price, composed of hard work and sacrifice. Sacrifices made of sleepless nights where I still decided to train in the morning, avoid eating pizza, skip a birthday cake slice and force myself to plan ahead the meals of the week. Motivation, commitment and sacrifices because I love myself. With time the sacrifices become lighter to handle and for me they become a healthy way of living, falling into the daily routine.

I knew before starting this journey that brought me to be a triathlete that nothing is given. I have built my character with determination and strong willingness to succeed.

THE IMPORTANCE OF ACTIVITY

Why do I feel better when I'm active? When I practice sports my body responds better to insulin, and managing glucose is easier. The logic behind is that when I exercise more, I need more energy, which mostly comes from using glucose. This means that my body becomes more sensitive to insulin, so I need less of it to control my blood sugar levels. On the other hand, when I'm not very active, things change. Not moving for a long time can make me more resistant to insulin, which means my cells don't respond to insulin as efficiently.

Being less insulin sensitive means that my body needs more insulin to keep my blood sugar stable when I'm not active. Thanks to my

Biotechnology and Oncology background I started to deep dive into the biology mechanism behind insulin action and understanding why these changes in insulin sensitivity happen has helped me manage my diabetes better.

For the past two years, I've been studying how my blood sugar levels change throughout the day with and without exercise. I've been considering different variables that can have an incidence on my glucose. I have noticed that adopting a high or low carb diet has an impact. Different types of exercises, at different intensities and duration have an impact. In 2022, my blood sugar levels weren't terrible, but there was definitely room for improvement. My HbA1c was around 7.5 (55 mmoL/L) and I was taking around 4 units of insulin in the morning, 8 units for lunch, 8 units for dinner, and 24 units of long-lasting insulin. I always look for better results and how to improve my overall health, despite the data above not being bad I do not want to compromise for medium results when I can reach a top one!

After having completed my oncology master, I had all the scientific background needed to start exploring the science of my own body.

I was living in Amsterdam, in a small studio by myself at the edge of the city. Even though I was doing everything correctly, such as eating healthily and exercising three times a week, I wasn't seeing any better results. The feelings of frustration were all over me. Moreover, I was adjusting my insulin based on my glucose levels and carb intake, but something was still off. I decided to start by writing down my exercise routine for the week. In the beginning of this journey, I worked out 3 or 4 times a week for an hour each day. Keeping track of the exercise was for me the first step of awareness and the trigger for positive changes.

Nowadays, I try to train every day; if possible, twice a day with differences between workout types. One session a day for a cardio session, while the second one consists of a shorter strength training or stability/stretch session. Yes, it is a lot! Training takes time and commitment, but the benefit I noticed in my health pushes me to keep going.

When I had a fixed and perfected training plan, thanks to my triathlon coach, Jose Lonzano, I started keeping track, in a separate table, of my nutrition schedule. Of course, as a diabetic person I counted carbohydrates, but I was not logging the food every day, at every meal. It might seem extra work, at times boring, and to be fair to you, sometimes it is. Before logging my food, I had the feeling of having eaten not enough or too much without exactly knowing how much or what were the nutritional components at the end of the day.

Becoming aware of what nutrients are inside the food I eat was a key part of optimizing the diabetes process. Understanding the grams of protein, fats and carbs in each food empowered me to make sensible choices. After a couple of weeks, I had more control and awareness of my food. For myself, I created different meal options that I have described from 1 to 4.

I developed this meal structure based on previous various nutritionists' advice, to help me stabilize my blood sugar levels throughout the day. The plan consists of a low-carb diet that is high in fat and protein. Later in this book I will show the changes and optimization to my nutrition plan thanks to the help of my nutritionist.

My first goal was to lose a couple of kilograms to feel better while exercising. Although, starting the process I realized I was administering more insulin compared to what I really needed, often creating

Hypoglycemia. The second goal was to reduce the amount of insulin I was taking, stabilizing my glucose throughout the day. In time, I found that this diet was effective in lowering my insulin intake, leading to less hunger during the day, less chocolate cravings in the evening and a sense of tiredness in the afternoon.

The reason why I decided to reduce carbohydrates is because they have the biggest impact on blood sugar levels and require more insulin to process them. Moreover, sometimes I found myself overestimating the amount of insulin needed for the carbohydrates and as a consequence I was triggering the insulin response. Counting carbs in meals has limitations, as many patients struggle to reach their blood sugar targets. These limitations include estimating meal portions, carb ratios, food preparation, and timing of insulin doses before meals.

I have found that a low-carb diet helps prevent both underestimating and overestimating carb intake, reducing the risk of high or low blood sugar events. Moreover, I have tested on my body that a diet with lower cholesterol and protein content helps to stabilize blood sugar levels. To support my thesis many studies have shown that meals high in fat and protein are effective for managing diabetes.

I suggest modifying the traditional "diabetes plate" composed of a quarter of protein, vegetables and carbohydrates by reducing the amount of carbs to less than a quarter of that plate. After having applied this concept, I noticed a more consistent blood sugar level on my monitor, with fewer spikes and drops. In addition, my body became more sensitive to insulin.

Having a nutrition strategy in place, I could focus on optimizing my exercise schedule, adding volume, and differentiating the exercises.

DATE	LUNCH	EVENING (WINTER)	EVENING
MON	CORE	SPINNING	OUTDOOR BIKE
TUE	STRENGHT	SWIM	SWIM
WED	YOGA	SPINNING	INTERVAL RUN
THU	CORE	BOXING	OPEN WATER SWIM
FRI	RUN	SWIM	OPEN WATER SWIM
SAT		LONG BIKE	LONG BIKE
SUN		LONG SWIM	LONG RUN

The table shows my weekly sport routine. The table is divided into lunch exercises and evening exercises. The type of exercise differs between summer and winter. The duration of the exercises is specified while the intensity varies from moderate to intense.

Monday

- Lunch Time: Core Stability exercises lasting 30 minutes.
- Winter Evening: Attend a spinning class for 45 minutes.
- Summer Evening: Go for a 90-minute bike ride.

Tuesday

- Lunch Time: Leg Strength exercises for 30 minutes.
- Winter Evening: Participate in a 60-minute swim session.
- Summer Evening: Continue with a 60-minute swim session.

Wednesday

- Lunch Time: Stability exercises for 30 minutes.

- Winter Evening: Join a 45-minute spinning course.
- Summer Evening: Engage in 60 minutes of interval running.

Thursday

- Lunch Time: Core Stability exercises for 30 minutes.
- Winter Evening: Take part in a 45-minute boxing class.
- Summer Evening: Swim in open water for 60 minutes.

Friday

- Lunch Time: Go for a 30-minute run.
- Winter Evening: Swim for 60 minutes.
- Summer Evening: Swim in open water for 60 minutes.

Saturday

- Lunch Time: No scheduled exercise.
- Winter Evening: Enjoy a 90-minute bike ride indoors.
- Summer Evening: Enjoy a 90-minute bike ride.

Sunday

- Lunch Time: No scheduled exercise.
- Winter Evening: Swim for 60 minutes.
- Summer Evening: Running for 90 minutes.

MEAL	OPTION 1	OPTION 2	OPTION 3	OPTION 4
BREAKFAST 8:30AM	1 APPLE + 20G DARK CHOCOLATE	20G DARK CHOCOLATE + 2 EGGS	100G BREAD + GEL	SPINACH SALAD + 10G BLUBERRY
SNACK 10:30AM	1 MANDARIN	1 APPLE	HALF BANANA	HALF BANANA
LUNCH 13:00PM	100G BRESAOLA + 200G SALAD + NUTS	200G CARPACCIO + 200G VEGETABLES	3GGS + 120G BEANS	CAPRESE SALAD + 100G BREAD
SNACK 17:00PM	20G CHEESE + 20G HAM	20G NUTS	BREAD + OIL	45G MUESLI
DINNER 21:00 PM	150G COOKED SALMON + 200G VEGETABLES	100G SMOKED SALMON + AVOCADO	150G CHICKEN + 50G RICE	150G FISH + 80G BREAD + 1TBS OIL

This table describes my nutrition plan with four different variations. I was following this plan when I started writing this diary in 2021. This nutrition plan was shaped thanks to previous nutritionist suggestions and my personal experience.

Breakfast (8:30 am)

- **Option 1:** Start your day with a light and quick option – 1 apple paired with 20 g of 90% dark chocolate.
- **Option 2:** Enjoy 1 piece of 90% dark chocolate alongside scrambled eggs for a protein-rich start.
- **Option 3 (Sport):** Fuel up with 100 g of brown bread, a banana, and an energy gel for sustained energy.
- **Option 4:** A nutritious option with spinach salad and 10 blueberries.

Snack (10:30 am)

- **Option 1 & 2**: Choose between a mandarin or an apple for a simple, refreshing snack.
- **Option 3 & 4**: Opt for a kiwi or half a banana for a quick energy boost.

Lunch (1:00 pm)

- **Option 1**: Enjoy a balanced meal with 100 g of bresaola, a 200 g salad with 10 tomatoes, and 10 walnuts.
- **Option 2**: A hearty option of 150 g roast beef or carpaccio with salad, or a classic pomodoro and mozzarella combination.
- **Option 3 (Sport)**: A protein-packed lunch with 3 eggs and 1 piece of fruit.
- **Option 4**: Indulge in burrata with tomato and 100 g of bread for a flavorful and satisfying meal.

Dinner (9:00 pm)

- **Option 1**: A nutritious dinner with 200 g of steamed vegetables (broccoli) and 150 g of salmon.
- **Option 2**: Choose between shakshuka or 100 g of smoked salmon with an avocado salad for a fresh and healthy option.
- **Option 3 (Sport)**: Enjoy 150 g of chicken paired with 50 g of rice for a balanced post-exercise meal.
- **Option 4**: Opt for 150 g of cod or chicken cooked in an air fryer, served with a 200 g salad for a light yet satisfying dinner.

Optional Snack (5:00 pm)

- **Option 1**: Choose dark chocolate or a piece of fruit for a light snack.
- **Option 2**: Have 2 slices of brown bread.
- **Option 3**: Enjoy 2 slices of brown bread with a piece of parmigiano.
- **Option 4**: Nuts plus 50 g of prosciutto and add carbs before endurance activities for extra energy.

For insight, after focusing on my diet and exercise for a month, I noticed that I needed less insulin when eating the same amount of carbohydrates as before. Additionally, my blood sugar levels were more stable, and I didn't have to constantly check my glucose monitor. Before achieving a stable blood sugar level, thanks to diet and exercise, I used to correct more frequently high blood sugar events. Moreover, as I post reflection, often, I was correcting postprandial hyperglycemia too quickly without giving the insulin enough time to work. This was causing a rollercoaster of highs and lows.

My takeaway is that it's important to be patient and trust the process instead of constantly chasing after the perfect glucose level. Unfortunately, too many diabetic Instagram influencers want to show us that they have perfect glucose management, but apart from being a lie per se, this creates false expectation and stress on people like us who are really trying to find the best strategy.

After three months following the optimized diet and exercise schedule my HbA1c was 6% (42 mmoL/L) from 7.5%. The new insulin values were 2 units of insulin in the morning, 4 units for lunch, 4 units for dinner, and 20 units of long-lasting insulin. This was quite a reduction compared to my starting insulin doses!

MY INSULIN DECISIONS

Every day I need to make hundreds of decisions regarding what to eat, when and how much insulin to inject. I really do my best to keep the glucose inside the "range", although, in my case, this constant commitment and dedication could easily evolve into frustration.

The general guideline is to keep the glucose between 80 mg/dL and 130 mg/dL (4.4 to 7.2 mmoL/L). This is what I see as a "green zone" in my continuous glucose monitor (CGM) app screen. Together with my diabetologist, my time in range (TIR) was established as 70–180 mg/dL (3.9–10.0 mmoL/L). Practicing lots of sport, I prefer to be on the safe side, preventing hypoglycemia.

Now I want to talk about my experience with diabetes management, hypothyroidism, and sport. Before discussing the strategies I use to manage my insulin and blood sugar, I want to give you an overview of my daily diabetes management and what past experiences brought me here today.

I have had diabetes since 1999 and my parents were injecting insulin for me. At the age of five, I started injecting my belly, as it was the easiest area to reach. During my teenage years, a new diagnosis came, Hashimoto hypothyroidism. This means that my thyroid is functioning less than a normal one and probably will progressively decrease its functioning over time creating a metabolic dysfunction. This pathology makes me feel more tired and lethargic during the day. Another side effect is a lower metabolic rate, making me more prone to accumulate adipose tissue.

Since then, I have been treated with a daily pill but a malfunctioning thyroid impacted my diabetes management negatively. Therefore, for a couple of years I tried a Medtronic insulin pump before the existence of continuous glucose monitors. The pump was great in helping with diabetes management, although not so great for me as a triathlete, always swimming, showering and sweating a lot. The pump had many negative points for me: the plaster was not lasting properly, the cannula was often damaged because of the many trainings and I decided to stop after being frustrated for months. Now, I am back using the insulin pens, Fiasp and Tresiba, with a continuous glucose monitor.

My first CGM was freestyle libre 1. Afterwards, version two and finally version three came out on the market. I was not really satisfied with freestyle libre, and I requested to move to Dexcom G6 and now Dexcom G7. My opinion regarding the glucose monitors is very net and brutal. I experienced less accuracy in the readings from freestyle Libre 3 during sport compared to Dexcom G7. If you are wondering how I noticed this discrepancy is because for 10 days, I wore both types of sensors, each on my arms. During exercising I was checking with the blood test the glucose and I was comparing the results between glucose monitors. I am very grateful for the technology I have available, but I have learned not to fully rely on it as it might fail. Before making any insulin decision, I always check how I feel without only blindly relying on the data.

In my daily routine, I am very careful on my diet, calculating the carbohydrates carefully trying to minimize insulin doses and injection times, as it becomes easier to track the active insulin in my body, preventing hypoglycemic events.

I will try to explain how I use the insulin during the day, when I decide to inject or when to integrate with sugar in a simple way. I consider it fundamental to measure the glucose before eating to decide the right amount of insulin depending on the food (amount of carbohydrates) I want to eat. The general rule is in case of hypoglycemia the integration is 15 grams of fast carbohydrates then wait for 15 minutes and if the glucose is stable integrate with a long lasting carbohydrate.

It becomes more complex if physical activity is involved, as usually I need to keep integrating during the physical activity and correct any hypoglycemia with extra long lasting carbohydrates. More details will be explained in detail later in this book. Following the guideline I follow regarding blood sugar and exercise.

SUGAR LEVEL	MG/DL	ACTION	SPORT IN THE NEXT HOUR
HIGH SUGAR LEVEL	>220-250	INSULIN	BIKE 50KM
ON TARGET SUGAR LEVEL	80-180	-	RUN 5KM
LOW SUGAR LEVEL	<80-50	SUGAR INTEGRATION	

This table describes my strategy to deal with nutrition integration and insulin with and without physical activity.

- **Very Low (<65 mg/dL):** If blood sugar levels are very low, it is crucial to consume 15 grams of simple (fast-acting) carbohydrates to quickly raise the levels, followed by 20 grams of long-lasting carbohydrates to maintain the level. Physical activity should be avoided until blood sugar stabilizes.
- **Low (<80-50 mg/dL):** Immediate intake of 15 grams of sugar is necessary to raise blood sugar levels. Add some carbohydrates if engaging in physical activity soon.

- **On Target (90-130 mg/dL):** Blood sugar levels are within the desired range, so no action is required. Physical activity can be performed without additional insulin.
- **Moderate (130-180 mg/dL):** Consuming 20 grams of long-lasting carbohydrates can help maintain blood sugar levels. Physical activity can be monitored without additional insulin.
- **High (>220-250 mg/dL):** Insulin administration is recommended to lower high blood sugar levels. Avoid physical activity until levels are brought under control.
- **Very High (>250 mg/dL):** Do not assume any carbohydrates as blood sugar levels are critically high. Physical activity is not recommended in this state.

Understanding the exact degree and way in which subjective carbohydrate expenditure is influenced in sports for a person with insulin-dependent diabetes is very complex, especially in team or long-term sports in which the energy metabolism involved varies enormously. After years of testing, data collection and I have found my strategy. The strategy was a long journey made mainly by mistakes because they are the ones that really made me learn. I would like to share my story and discovery strategy, to give my readers inspirations and tools to follow a similar thinking process.

OPTIMIZED SCHEDULE

My life with diabetes has been a rollercoaster of emotions, and acceptance has not always come easily. As an introverted kid, I have never talked about my chronic conditions to my friends. Carrying this weight on my shoulder became unbearable at some point in my life. After a year of struggling, denying my disease, and feeling alone and misunderstood by my family and friends, I needed a new challenge, moving to Amsterdam. This radical change in lifestyle and daily routine was a real test. It also forced me to change my main language, change eating habits, change diabetologists, switch healthcare systems, and adapt to a new glucose measurement unit—from mg/dL to mmoL/L. Throwing myself into the unknown was scary, but I want to share the positive message I learnt. Everything is possible, even with Diabetes.

Throughout this journey, and as I recount in this diary, I started recording my values in mg/dL before shifting to mmoL/L, as imposed by the Dutch healthcare system. For clarity, I have included the conversion in the following table.

mmoL/L	mg/dL	mmoL/L	mg/dL
2.2	40	10	180
3.3	60	11.1	200
4.4	80	12.5	225
5.5	100	13.9	250
6.7	120	15	270
7.8	140	16.6	300
8.9	160	20	360

This table provides a conversion from millimoles per liter (mmoL/L) to milligrams per deciliter (mg/dL), commonly used in blood glucose monitoring. This table helps to quickly convert blood glucose readings from mmoL/L to mg/dL or vice versa.

Getting the right balance of sports, food, and insulin is crucial for effective diabetes management. Through careful tracking and adjustments, I have managed to significantly increase my time in range, reducing my insulin intake, leading to better overall health and control of my blood sugar levels.

Insulin management is a cornerstone of diabetes care. Proper dosing ensures that blood sugar levels remain within target ranges, preventing hyperglycemia (high blood sugar) and hypoglycemia (low blood sugar). According to a study by Choudhary et al. (2016), personalized insulin dosing, when combined with continuous glucose monitoring and regular physical activity, can significantly improve glycemic control, and reduce the incidence of hypoglycemia.

Adjusting insulin dosage based on activity levels and dietary intake can help in achieving better diabetes control. Studies have shown that engaging in regular physical activity can enhance insulin sensitivity, reducing the amount of insulin required to maintain normal blood glucose levels. Similarly, strategic eating patterns, such as incorporating low glycemic index foods and balanced meals, can minimize blood sugar spikes and lower insulin needs.

At this point all this work consisting of tracking the food and planning exercise might sound silly to you, or just a lot of work. Well, I am not going to lie, it really is, and the best part is that the work is not over yet. As depicted in the following table, after developing a tailored exercise and nutrition plan, I have optimized my insulin regimen to manage my diabetes more effectively. This is my final suggestion to optimize the overall diabetes management, reflecting on your day-to-day values. This insulin scheme was achieved through consistent adjustments and careful monitoring during 2022-23.

INSULIN INTAKE	UNITS	INSULIN TYPE
BREAKFAST	0	
LUNCH	2-4	FIASP
DINNER	2-4	FIASP
BEFORE BED	14-10	TRESIBA

The table shows the number of insulin injections during the day, with the amount (units) and insulin type. This insulin plan is what I have reached during 2022-23 thanks to optimized training and nutrition plan.

The previous table outlines my current insulin regimen, which I have fine-tuned through the year to balance my blood glucose levels effectively. The reduction in insulin dosage reflects my improved insulin sensitivity and control achieved through daily physical activity and a carefully managed diet. While I'm pleased with my progress, I continue to seek ways to further optimize my insulin usage. The goal is to use even less insulin by refining my diet and adjusting exercise routines.

Research indicates that adopting a low-carbohydrate diet can lead to a further reduction in insulin requirements. Despite this evidence, I do not follow a low-carbohydrate diet but a balanced one where my intake of carbohydrates is smart and planned according to physical activity. Moreover, high-intensity interval training (HIIT) has been shown to improve insulin sensitivity, potentially reducing insulin needs. Endurance sports such as triathlon showed me to have similar effects in improving insulin sensitivity. Therefore, my intention for this new year is to keep my motivation high and be focused on improving even more my general health and diabetes management. Because, hey, if not now, when?

Reducing insulin intake is not only about lowering medication doses but also about improving metabolic health and reducing the risk of insulin resistance. High levels of insulin over time can contribute to insulin resistance, a condition where the body's cells become less responsive to insulin, necessitating higher doses to control blood sugar.

Today, after one year of following a smart low carb diet and exercising every day, together with a daily attention on my lifestyle choices, my HbA1c (Average Blood Sugar Level) is 6% and I am injecting around 0-2 units of insulin in the morning, 2-4 units for lunch, 2-4 units for dinner, and 14 units of long-lasting insulin.

In the next chapter, I will explore how insulin works, the mechanisms of insulin resistance, and strategies to overcome this challenge.

7. INSULIN MECHANISMS

My background as a biotechnology scientist and oncology master graduated scientist focused my attention on the deep mechanism of cell metabolism. The cells use sugar to generate energy, but excessive sugar intake can lead to conditions such as diabetes and potentially increase the risk of cancer through mechanisms like increased insulin levels, inflammation and altered cell metabolism.

During my studies I have learned how both cancer and diabetes involve significant changes in how cells process glucose, impacting overall health. I remember how I was diving into anatomy, physiology and biochemistry books with passion and dedication. My drive was pushing me to stay up till midnight in the library to study and meet aspirant doctors' colleagues to exchange opinions and ideas, dreaming about a future where diabetes could be only an old memory.

I graduated in Oncology at the University of Amsterdam, with distinction. Diabetes and cancer have in common the use of glucose; therefore, I will mention how the cells use it in the biological process. Cells use glucose as a primary source of energy. The process involves several key steps, that are important to know to deeply understand how as diabetes patients we can improve our condition:

- **Glucose Uptake:** Glucose enters cells through specific transport proteins on the cell membrane, such as GLUT transporters.
- **Glycolysis:** Once inside, glucose is broken down in the cytoplasm through glycolysis, producing pyruvate and a small amount

of ATP (energy).

- **Cellular Respiration:** Pyruvate is then transported into the mitochondria, where it is further processed in the Krebs cycle to generate more ATP, releasing carbon dioxide and water as waste products. If oxygen is scarce, pyruvate can be converted into lactate instead (fermentation).

This process of converting glucose into energy is crucial for all cell functions, from growth and division to repair and communication. Although this process of converting glucose into energy is not possible if insulin is not present as in Diabetes T1.

Type 1 diabetes (T1D) is an autoimmune condition characterized by pancreatic beta cell destruction, absolute insulin deficiency, and impaired glucose metabolism. The following explanation of how insulin works in our cells is a technical explanation taken from a scientific article as I believe in the importance of deeply understanding the biological mechanism of our body.

Insulin is a peptide hormone released by islets of pancreatic beta cells. This hormone has significant effects on metabolic pathways, and thereby, it is critical for normal homeostasis of the body metabolism. Any defect in these pathways may lead to impaired insulin-dependent glucose entering the cells, known as insulin resistance in adipocytes and skeletal muscles.

The following figure shows how the insulin signal transduction starts by binding insulin to the α chain of insulin receptor (IR), which is a transmembrane tyrosine kinase composed of two chains as α and β. This process stimulates autophosphorylation in the β chain, which in turn recruits different adaptor proteins such as IRSs (insulin receptor substrates), Shc protein (SHC-transforming), and APS protein (adapter protein with a PH and SH2 domain).

These events provide a suitable binding site for IRS-1 (insulin receptor substrate-1) and activate it, which links to PI3K (phosphoinositide 3-kinase) and catalyzes the conversion of PIP2 (phosphatidylinositol 4,5-bisphosphate) to PIP3 (phosphatidylinositol 3,4,5-trisphosphate). In addition, PIP3 is itself a potent activator for PKB (protein kinase B, also known as Akt), which facilitates glucose entering the cells by localization of GLUT-4 (glucose transporter type 4) (J Diabetes Res. 2021).

Insulin is a great hormone! Insulin binds its receptor and allows glucose to enter the cell, giving us the energy to be active. Every time I dive deep into the biological mechanism of our body I am mesmerized about how we are able to perform such complex processes and how easily we fall down sick from a small virus.

Coming back to our hormone, Insulin. Despite Insulin being a good hormone, the insulin *response* is the bad guy, and I will explain why.

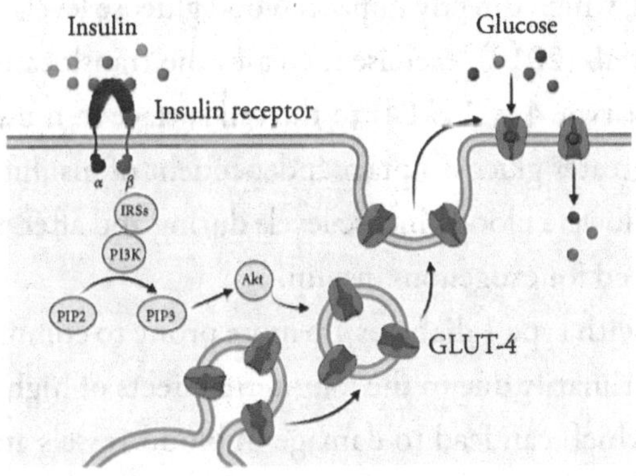

The figure shows how insulin acts via complicated sequential steps known as insulin signal transduction (IST). (J Diabetes Res. 2021)

INSULIN RESPONSE

Insulin is a great hormone, which is impossible to live without. However, the insulin *response* is not so great.

Insulin helps to lower blood glucose. For example, if a person with diabetes has a blood glucose value of 300 mg/dL (15.5 mmoL/L) and will inject 2 units of insulin, the glucose will drop to, for example, 100 mg/dL (5.5 mmoL/L). How and where did that 200 mg/dL difference go? Insulin takes what we are not burning, for instance our 200 mg/dL and puts it into storage, named fat. This is called insulin response, and I will call it "The Bad Guy" as the Huberman Lab mentions in his podcast.

Regular physical activity significantly influences how our body manages glucose and insulin. Research has shown that when we engage in exercise, our muscles become more effective at clearing glucose from the bloodstream, leading to more stable blood glucose levels and reduced insulin requirements. Physical activity enhances glucose uptake by muscles, which directly impacts blood glucose levels. According to Colberg et al. (2010), exercise increases the translocation of glucose transporter type 4 (GLUT4) to the cell surface in muscle tissues, facilitating greater glucose uptake independent of insulin. This process effectively lowers blood glucose levels during and after exercise, reducing the need for exogenous insulin.

People with type 1 diabetes are more prone to complications such as stroke primarily due to the long-term effects of high blood glucose levels, which can lead to damage in blood vessels and contribute to the development of atherosclerosis. This condition, characterized by the buildup of fatty deposits in the arteries, can restrict blood flow to the brain, increasing the risk of stroke. Additionally, individuals with type 1 diabetes often experience other related health issues, such as hypertension and dyslipidemia, which further elevates stroke risk.

Diabetes complications could be prevented with a healthy lifestyle, personalised diet and training schedule, closely monitored by health care specialists. Sport and nutrition are key to prevent insulin resistance and increase good cardiovascular functionalities. Moreover, a healthy lifestyle decreases body inflammation, decreasing ROS (reactive species of oxygen) and promoting the good health of mitochondria.

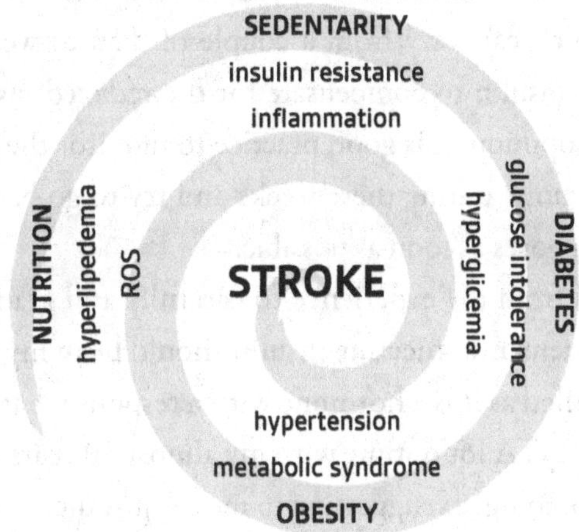

The figure shows the link between nutrition, sedentarity and Diabetes. The complications could be prevented with a healthy lifestyle that includes balanced nutrition, physical activity and good diabetes management.

I do not take my insulin decisions lightly, as in the long term could impact my overall well being. I try, together with the expert, to perfect my insulin dosage, to avoid in the first instance hypoglycemia and hyperglycemia events, and prevent diabetes complications due to the insulin response.

INSULIN RESISTANCE

Insulin resistance is a condition in which the body's cells don't respond effectively to insulin, so they don't take in glucose as efficiently. I have experienced it multiple times for various reasons such as sicknesses, high stress or menstrual cycle. During these insulin resistant periods, which can vary from a couple of days to weeks, I need to inject more insulin to compensate for the reduced insulin effectiveness. In my opinion, it is good practice to monitor the glucose values and insulin units during these weeks and try to go back to the standard insulin doses as soon as possible.

I learned from my experience to carefully and gradually increase my insulin demand. Injecting insulin should be in my opinion more dose controlled as it is a hormone with a response that it is named as "The Bad Guy". A lot of time with my almost 30 years with Diabetes I heard diabetologists suggesting to me to "just increase the doses". Is this a healthy approach? Of course, it is important to make sure the glucose comes back in range, but what is the other side of the coin? Perhaps, together with the advice to increase the doses, we should also increase physical activity or reduce the sugar or carbohydrate intake. Unfortunately, I understand it takes more will power and effort to avoid eating something we like instead of increasing a couple of units the injection we would have done anyway, although, I am still wondering, if this should be the advice in the first place. Regarding this topic, I will share my story.

At first, I was not paying much attention to my insulin doses and over time, my body adapted to the higher insulin demand, starting the process of storing body fat mass. During this period, I was suffering from stomach disorders and muscle pain, gaining more and more weight over time. I could feel my abdominal fat tissue was increasing, feeling more swollen and inflamed. I looked up some articles and as I suspected, the adipose tissue is an active endocrine organ that produces various signaling molecules, known as adipokines.

Changes in the secretion of these adipokines can influence inflammation and metabolic health. It is shown that Adiponectin, an adipokine with anti-inflammatory properties, is often found in lower levels in individuals with type 1 and 2 diabetes.

After reading this, a change in my mindset happened, and I have decided to commit to try to fight this chronic inflammation as much as possible, by having a healthy lifestyle. This means a healthy diet, avoiding processed food and refined sugar and high amounts of carbohydrates, if not needed by the body. Moreover, I always try to keep myself moving at least one or two hours every day.

As a summary, I have concluded that insulin resistance impacts the way the body stores and utilizes fat. Increased insulin levels may promote fat storage, particularly in adipose tissue. Adipose tissue creates inflammation, promoting insulin resistance mechanisms.

I experience firsthand that with diabetes, insulin resistance could contribute to higher blood sugar levels, making it more challenging to manage the condition. Lifestyle changes, such as regular exercise and a healthy diet, can help improve insulin sensitivity, reducing therefore the amount of insulin, body inflammation and body fat mass.

8. CARBOHYDRATES

I was 10 years old when my diabetologist decided I was ready to start carbohydrate counting. Before, from the age of three to ten, my parents took care of most of the decisions. In 1999, diabetes was managed differently, so please do not be surprised if I did not have an insulin pump right from the start or I was not able to count carbohydrates.

At the time, I did not know what the doctor was going to tell me, and she planned a meeting that seemed very serious and revolutionary for my diabetes management. In the hospital, the seriousness in the room was palpable. The doctor handed me a little book with figures of food, such as plates of pasta, rice or polenta in different sizes: small, medium, and large. Each figure in the book had a specified amount of carbohydrates in grams, allowing a quick understanding of how much insulin would have been required. On the side, we made a brief calculation to understand how much insulin I would require for 10 grams of carbohydrates, essentially determining my insulin-to-carb ratio.

At the time, my insulin-to-carb ratio was 1 unit for every 10 grams of carbohydrates (1:10). This ratio is something that can change over time; for instance, mine changed to 2:10 during high school and came back to 1:10 during university. Nowadays, my insulin to carbohydrates ratio is 1:20 grams. Understanding the number of grams of carbohydrates in different foods is helpful for making the right decisions about insulin amounts. However, as I walked out of that hospital room, I immediately understood that this knowledge alone was not enough to achieve good diabetes management.

Nowadays, carbohydrates are a fundamental component of my diet with sport and play a significant role in glucose stability for me as an individual with type 1 diabetes and as an athlete. Although I do not abuse food rich in carbohydrates, I carefully plan my meals depending on physical activity. Understanding how each macronutrient is digested and processed into energy is key to mastering diabetes. Carbohydrate metabolism has a huge effect on blood sugar levels and dictates insulin demand, as carbohydrates are the main component requiring insulin.

When I consume foods rich in carbohydrates, my digestive system breaks them down into simpler sugars, such as glucose. Glucose is then absorbed into my bloodstream, causing blood sugar levels to rise. Through understanding the science behind fat, protein, and carbohydrates, and with my experience, I have mastered how to dose them properly throughout the day depending on physical activity.

My approach towards carbohydrates could seem controversial but honestly it really works for my body and my diabetes combined with hypothyroidism. My strategy is to eat carbohydrates when the body needs them, such as to fuel a long aerobic activity or a race or to recover from a big effort. I managed to get rid of carbohydrates in any other circumstances that are not the times when my body needs them. In practice I eat carbohydrates when I am about to burn them as fuel, avoiding injecting more insulin to manage them.

Now I can say I do not miss them at all. I do not deny the strong willpower that I need to use, to skip some bread near the main meals, avoid snacks and pass on pizza nights. The benefit of saying "No" and going for a different option such as protein shakes, vegetables snacks, has so many positive effects on my mind and body that it is not difficult anymore. This different approach towards carbohydrates helps me avoid hyperglycemia and unnecessary insulin amounts. As I mentioned before, I do not follow a ketogenic diet, but I balance my carbohydrates carefully.

By using this approach, it is fundamental to understand how different carbohydrates get absorbed by our bodies and the differences between simple and complex, which I will explain in the next section.

MINDFUL CARBOHYDRATES

In the context of type 1 diabetes, managing blood sugar levels is an ongoing challenge. Carbohydrates can serve as a valuable tool for stabilizing glucose. When consumed in the right amounts and in a controlled, predictable manner, carbohydrates can be matched with insulin doses. This approach, often referred to as carbohydrate counting, helps individuals with type 1 diabetes, including myself, keep their blood sugar levels within a target range. By understanding the carbohydrate content of foods and calculating the corresponding insulin dose, it becomes easier to manage the post-meal rise in blood sugar.

A key element in carbohydrate management is differentiating between simple and complex carbohydrates, as they have different glycemic indexes. Simple carbohydrates are sugars with uncomplicated chemical structures, such as fructose and glucose. When I consume simple carbs, they quickly turn into sugar in my bloodstream, causing my blood sugar levels to skyrocket. This unpredictability can make managing diabetes a daily challenge if simple carbs are consumed alone, meaning not together with protein or fats, and not at the appropriate moment.

Complex carbohydrates are the slow and steady players. They consist of longer chains of sugars, like those found in whole grains, fruits, and vegetables. This slow and steady release is a blessing because it helps me maintain more stable blood sugar levels. I know that when I choose complex carbs, I'm less likely to experience those sudden spikes and crashes. From scientific literature it is proved that complex carbohydrates are fundamental during endurance sports, and I do make use of them to face my aerobic endurance workout.

Understanding the glycemic index has been a game-changer in my life with type 1 diabetes. It's like having a secret code to decipher how different carbs will affect my blood sugar. The glycemic index measures how quickly a carbohydrate-containing food raises blood sugar. Low-GI foods are my friends because they cause a slow and controlled increase in my blood sugar levels. On the other hand, high-GI foods are like the speed bumps I want to avoid because they lead to rapid spikes. By using the glycemic index, I can make more informed choices about what I eat, aiming for stability and predictability in my blood sugar levels.

Many factors can affect a food's glycemic index, including the following:

- **Processing:** Grains that have been refined—removing the bran and the germ—have a higher glycemic index than minimally processed whole grains.
- **Physical form:** Finely ground grain is more rapidly digested than coarsely ground grain. This is why eating whole grains in

their "whole form" like brown rice, or oats can slow the rate of digestion and cause a more gradual and lower rise in blood sugar.

- **Fiber content:** High-fiber foods don't contain as much digestible carbohydrate, so it slows the rate of digestion and causes a more gradual and lower rise in blood sugar.
- **Ripeness:** Ripe fruits and vegetables tend to have a higher glycemic index than un-ripened fruit.
- **Fat content and acid content:** Meals with fat or acid are converted more slowly into sugar.

I started empowering myself with all the information I could find, reading books and scientific articles about nutrition and diabetes type 1. I found it useful to look at some graphs of an Instagram influencer; She calls herself the Glucose Goddess.

The Glucose Goddess, also known as Jessie Inchauspé, is an Instagram influencer and biochemist who focuses on educating people about the effects of glucose on overall health. Her main concept revolves around the idea that by understanding and managing blood glucose levels, individuals can improve their energy, mood, weight, and long-term health. She shares practical tips on how to flatten glucose spikes through diet and lifestyle changes, such as eating foods in a specific order, combining certain nutrients to minimize glucose fluctuations, and timing meals strategically.

Sharing my story and mentioning the glucose goddess has the purpose of making scientific knowledge accessible and actionable for a general audience, emphasizing the importance of stable glucose levels for optimal health.

Jessie, not affected by Diabetes, started looking at how food changes her blood sugar, as us with Diabetes know, some foods are really creating huge spikes compared to others depending on the Glycemic Index. After being inspired by her work, I also tried to replicate her graphs looking at how different types of food influence the blood glucose. The difference between us is that I have Type 1 Diabetes.

I want to summarize here the impact of different foods on blood glucose levels by emphasizing the importance of food order, combinations, and timing.

- **Food Order:** Eating vegetables and proteins before carbohydrates can significantly reduce glucose spikes, as fiber and proteins slow down the absorption of sugars.

- **Food Combinations:** Pairing carbohydrates with healthy fats, fiber, and proteins helps mitigate glucose spikes. For example, adding avocado or nuts to a carb-rich meal can stabilize blood sugar levels.

- **Timing and Portions:** Consuming smaller portions of carbohydrates and avoiding sugary snacks on an empty stomach can prevent sharp glucose increases.

By following these principles, I tried myself, I could maintain more stable glucose levels, leading to improved energy, reduced cravings, better mood, and overall health benefits.

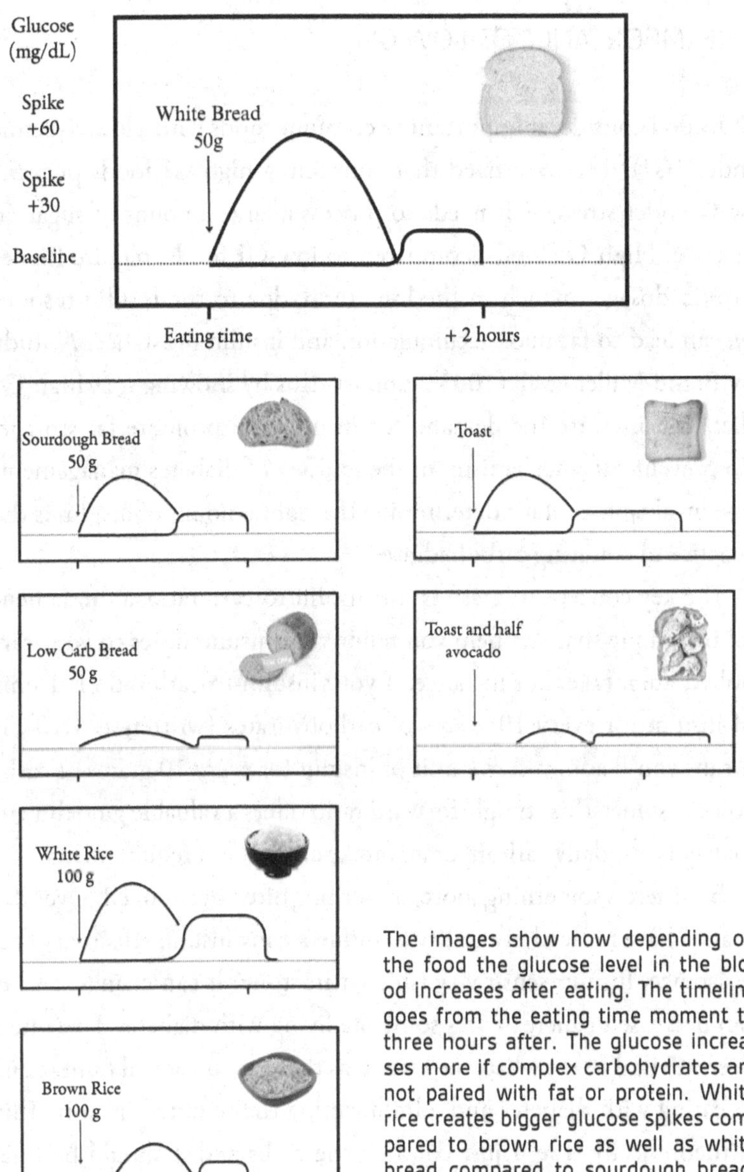

The images show how depending on the food the glucose level in the blood increases after eating. The timeline goes from the eating time moment to three hours after. The glucose increases more if complex carbohydrates are not paired with fat or protein. White rice creates bigger glucose spikes compared to brown rice as well as white bread compared to sourdough bread, same for a plain toast compared to an avocado toast.

THE IMPORTANCE OF LOW GI

Why do I consider it important to consume foods with a low glycemic index (GI)? I have noticed that consuming high-GI foods puts my body under stress, as it needs to process a large amount of sugar all at once. High-GI foods, compared to low-GI foods, require higher insulin dosages, which in the long term, due to the insulin response, can lead to fat mass accumulation and insulin resistance. A study by Brand-Miller et al. (2003) supports this by showing that high-GI diets can increase the demand for insulin and promote fat storage. To prevent this mechanism, in the journey of diabetes management, one invaluable tool for determining the right amount of insulin is the practice of counting carbohydrates.

The key concept to grasp is the insulin-to-carb ratio, a fundamental technique that can help you tailor your insulin doses to your carbohydrate intake. For instance, if your insulin-to-carb ratio is 1 unit of insulin for every 10 grams of carbohydrates (written as 1:10), it means you'll administer 1 unit of insulin for every 10 grams of carbs you consume. This straightforward ratio offers a valuable guideline to manage your daily carbohydrate intake and insulin requirements.

But there's something more, something often overlooked. Over the years, I have noticed my ability to influence my insulin sensitivity and resistance. Insulin sensitivity isn't set in stone; it can change, and it can decrease or increase. As someone living with diabetes, I've often been advised to eat whatever I want, as there are no actual limitations in eating with diabetes and administering the required insulin. This is theoretically true. I just counted the carbs and it should be fine. However, the reality is that when diabetes became a part of my life, my approach to food evolved. It's not just about counting carbs; it's about embracing a holistic perspective on nutrition.

According to a study by Wang et al. (2013), lifestyle interventions, including diet and physical activity, significantly impact insulin sensitivity. This means that by making informed dietary choices and incorporating regular exercise, I can actively improve my insulin sensitivity, reduce insulin resistance, and better manage my diabetes. This holistic approach to nutrition goes beyond just calculating insulin dosages based on carbohydrate intake; it involves understanding how different foods affect my body and using this knowledge to maintain optimal metabolic health.

This mind and behavioral shift played a crucial role in my life. I promised myself to avoid any possible future development of insulin resistance. In my own journey, I've observed changes in my insulin-to-carb ratio over the years. Now, I am proud to say I am very close to my best diabetes management. This journey isn't just about adapting my eating habits but also enhancing my mindset. Us all with diabetes, seek a balance between living a normal life, enjoying food, while recognizing that stricter dietary rules sometimes need to be our companion.

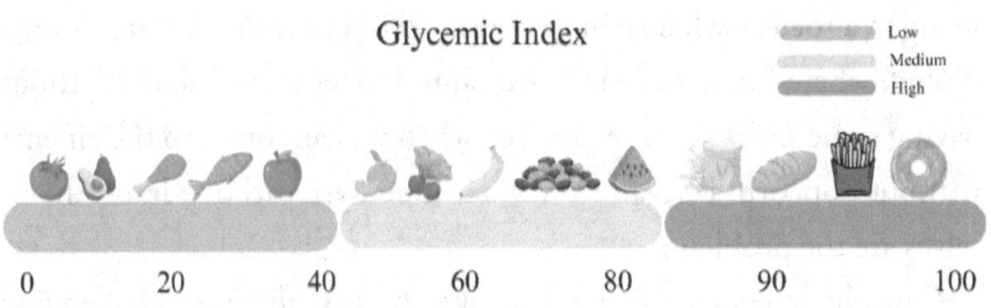

The figure shows the glycemic index (GI) for starches, vegetables, fruits, proteins, and dairy.

My learning from this nutritional journey was that achieving good diabetes control is not about full restriction or following any fancy diet or exercising all day long, but it is about finding a routine that makes sense for me.

Understanding my needs and discovering how my body works and reacts to certain food is something that I need to be aware of to take a step forward towards better diabetes management.

MY REFLECTION

Carbohydrates, depending on their type, create different glucose spikes curves. Becoming aware of the nutritional components and their effects it's extremely important in the journey of mastering diabetes management. My first step was selecting carbohydrates with a low glycemic index (GI). As a result, I noticed an improvement in my glucose level stability as well as a reduction in insulin requirements. A study by Jenkins et al. (2002) supports this, showing that low-GI diets improve blood glucose control and reduce insulin demands. However, I began to question if our use of carbohydrates is excessive. We are living in a society where a huge consumption of carbohydrates is promoted, where for some reason we cannot meet some friends without having some snacks on the table, or when we cannot go to the cinema without popcorn. I began to wonder if perhaps carbohydrates themselves are the problem.

Carbohydrates are the nutrients which cause the most challenging glucose spikes, which lead to the need for more insulin, resulting in glucose instability and more frequent episodes of hyperglycemia or hypoglycemia. This cycle of glucose spikes and subsequent insulin surges can disrupt my ability to maintain steady blood sugar levels and increase the risk of both high and low blood glucose episodes. Therefore, managing carbohydrate intake is crucial, but it is equally important to consider the type and quality of carbohydrates consumed to achieve optimal glucose control.

Carbohydrates have the highest impact on blood sugar because they require the most insulin. Currently, the common way to manage meals high in carbohydrates is through carbohydrate counting. However, this method has many limitations, as it is shown that patients often do not manage to reach their targets. I, too, often struggle to maintain my glucose levels within the desired range when consuming a meal reach of carbohydrates.

The limitations of carbohydrate counting include the estimation of meal portions, the carb ratio that changes depending on food preparation, and selecting the timing of pre-prandial bolus. Therefore, I started following a low-carb diet to avoid underestimating or overestimating carbohydrate content in meals, which reduces the chances of hyperglycemia and hypoglycemia events.

For me, with diabetes T1 and hypothyroidism, a diet with a reduced amount of carbohydrates, low in cholesterol and high in protein is the way to achieve glucose stability. My use of carbohydrates is not abolished, on the contrary it is controlled and planned in a smart way, depending on the body's needs.

If no physical activity is involved, I propose a change to the classical diabetes plate, reducing the amount of carbohydrates to less than a quarter of the plate, rather than a full quarter every meal. My approach towards carbohydrates is not demonizing them but using them as an important source of energy when my body needs them to face sport. Rather than eliminating them entirely, such as a ketogenic diet, I make conscious choices of my carbohydrates intake and timing.

Every diet and exercise plan should be shaped based on individual needs consulting and healthcare professionals.

9. MY NUTRITION PLAN

During my childhood, every six months, I had a day-long hospital visit that included a blood exam, thyroid echography, and appointments with the diabetologist and nutritionist doctors. I remember these days as very stressful because they were long and often painful. My mom always wanted to arrive at the hospital as early as possible, get the blood exam done, and then wait for the doctors to call us for the appointment. In the pediatric hospital, sometimes there were volunteers who made us draw and color, which made a huge difference for me. I don't remember the stress of the day; I only remember the joy of going home with my homemade puppet picture.

However, when I grew up and moved to the teenage section, there were no fun activities anymore—I just had to endure it. After a long boring morning, finally, the nutritionist called my name. As I entered the room, the nurses started measuring my height and weight. Afterwards, we reviewed my daily nutrition. I will always remember the first question she asked and her initial advice: "What do you eat for breakfast?" "A toast." "Keep going with a toast."

Probably, there was nothing inherently wrong with toast. However, I expected more from the nutritionists I encountered. I wanted some education and a personalized nutrition plan tailored to my body type and activity profile. Moreover, I hoped she would have guided me towards optimizing my nutrition, as I was already part of a competitive swimming team at the time. Through my journey with diabetes,

I learned to answer the nutrition questions and understand my body needs by myself.

What is my approach to nutrition with diabetes? First, I adopt a balanced diet, which is crucial for overall health and provides the body with essential nutrients in the right proportions. A balanced diet has been shown to support effective diabetes management by improving glycemic control and reducing the risk of complications. For example, a study by Franz et al. (2002) found that dietary interventions focusing on balanced nutrition, including the appropriate proportions of carbohydrates, proteins, and fats, significantly improved blood glucose levels and overall health outcomes in individuals with diabetes. The key nutritional components to include in a balanced diet are five plus water:

- **Proteins** in meat, poultry, fish, eggs, dairy, legumes, and nuts. They are essential for building and repairing tissues.
- **Carbohydrates** can be obtained from grains, fruits, vegetables, and legumes. They are the body's primary energy source.
- **Fats:** Healthy fats come from sources like avocados, nuts, seeds, and olive oil. They support cell structure, hormone production, and nutrient absorption.
- **Vitamins and Minerals:** Obtained from a variety of fruits, vegetables, whole grains, and lean proteins. They play crucial roles in various bodily functions.
- **Fiber** is found in fruits, vegetables, whole grains, and legumes. It aids digestion, promotes a feeling of fullness, and supports heart health.
- **Hydration:** Water is essential for overall health, regulating body temperature, aiding digestion, and supporting various physiological processes.

CALORIES CALCULATOR

After identifying the key nutrients, I needed to determine the appropriate proportions to eat. This involves estimating the number of calories needed per day, considering factors such as age, gender, weight, height, activity level, and overall health goals. An easy way to do this is by using available online tools to calculate daily calorie needs.

An assessment of energy needs is a vital component in the development and continual evaluation of an effective nutrition plan. This calorie calculator is an invaluable tool to calculate the number of calories I should eat per day, aligned to my age, height, gender, weight, activity levels and (importantly) my weight/fitness goals.

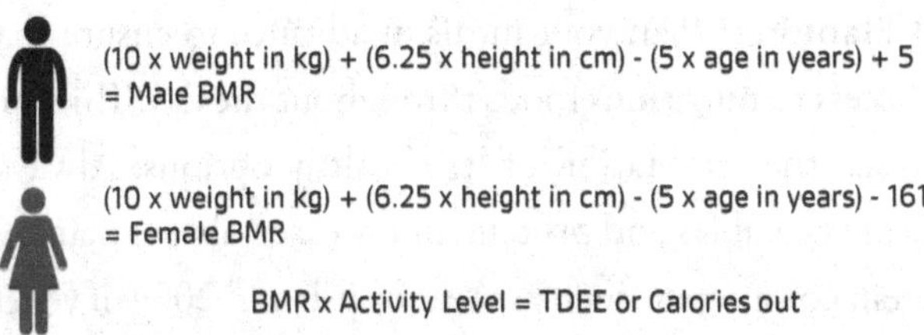

The figure shows how to calculate the "calory out" given the basal metabolic rate (BMR) and activity level.

Having an idea of the nutritional needs for my diet is the foundation for creating and following a nutrition plan. Thanks to the help of my nutritionist, I started following a structured food plan. This nutrition scheme specifies what I need to eat and when, detailing the amounts in grams of carbs, protein, and fats after every meal and the total calories per day.

Having a nutrition plan offers several benefits, including meeting nutrient requirements, managing weight, and improving physical performance while maintaining good mental health. My goal with the diet was to get in perfect shape for the triathlon racing season.

Changing my nutrition habits is a difficult task, and sticking to a plan instead of spontaneity can be challenging for someone often not so organized like me. In my experience, it is often difficult to follow a plan, which is why I would like you to consider the following tips:

- **Set Realistic Goals:** Establish achievable and realistic nutritional goals. Sometimes a small action, that is almost silly not to do, is better than a bigger one. This will help in introducing a new routine to your life, changing the bad habits.

- **Meal Planning:** Plan your meals in advance to ensure that you have access to nutritious foods throughout the day. This can help you resist the temptation of less healthy options. Always plan meals of vegetables and protein, in my case I always plan 100g of a protein component such as meat or fish and 200g of vegetables on the side.

- **Preparation is Key:** Prepare healthy snacks and meals in advance to make it easier to stick to your plan, especially when you're busy. In my case, I like boiling 6 eggs in advance and storing them in the fridge. In this way I have a protein snack ready, avoiding the temptation of chocolate and biscuits.

- **Portion Control:** Be mindful of portion sizes to avoid overeating. My tips are to use smaller plates and bowls to help with portion control. Moreover, try to be mindful while eating, be focused and present in the moment, enjoying your meal.

- **Track Your Progress:** Keep a food diary or use mobile apps to track your food intake and monitor your progress. This can help you stay accountable and identify areas for improvement. Using the Dexcom or Freestyle app for adding notes on your food and activity is an easy option! I use an app called Lifesum, giving me insight into the carbs, protein, and fat percentage of an ingredient. Give me meal suggestions depending on my kind of diet.

Remember that flexibility is key, and it's okay to enjoy treats in moderation. The goal is to establish sustainable, healthy eating habits that align with my lifestyle.

One of my main objectives is to allow younger people to face challenges with greater awareness of nutrition and sport. I would like to be present, listen and encourage by donating my tools and share my experience acquired in my daily management.

FOLLOWING A NUTRITION PLAN

During my 27 years with type 1 diabetes, I have consulted multiple nutritionists and dietologists. What I have learned is that your mindset is the most important influencer of whether a particular diet will be effective for you. The diet that reformed me came when I was ready for a change and ready to commit.

I went to many nutritionists thinking they would tell me something revolutionary, and every time that was not the case I was leaving with a bitter taste of disappointment. Then I realized: The change had to start within myself.

Finally, when I met my nutritionist in the Netherlands, I was ready mentally to commit and follow a structured plan. The nutrition plan helped me achieve better control of my diabetes levels. The first step I have introduced was the meal preparation. Despite my nature of being spontaneous and living day by day, I forced myself to be organized in my grocery shopping and meal preparation. Having fixed portions of food assists in counting carbohydrates and planning the right amount of insulin. I found this beneficial because it decreased glucose unpredictability caused by guessing insulin units, resulting in more stable glucose levels. Moreover, over time, having a structured plan leads to a reduction in the amount of insulin needed daily. For me, this was a great achievement! The reduction of insulin doses was the consequence of achieving more glucose stability avoiding hyperglycemia and hypoglycemia events. Overall meaning better glucose management decreasing the insulin response and insulin resistance.

In my diet, the day starts with a good breakfast! Eating breakfast is a must; it gives me energy and makes me feel full, preventing a huge sense of hunger by lunchtime. I usually opt for a savory breakfast as I noticed this helps prevent glucose spikes. My three simple breakfasts are:

- 3 scrambled eggs with a cappuccino;
- 30g of chicken and 30g of cheese on a toast, with the option to add an egg;
- 200g of natural yogurt with 30g of nuts.

Combining protein with carbs helps my glucose remain stable and provides a sense of satiety. Lunch and dinner follow the same principle: 80g to 150g of meat or fish with 200g of vegetables.

- Roast beef carpaccio.
- Grilled salmon with roasted vegetables.
- Chicken in the oven with vegetables.
- Omelette.

I have a lot of different options for these meals, but I will show a few examples that are very easy to prepare. Carpaccio is one of my favorites—very simple and low in fat—along with bresaola. Other options include an omelet with cheese or salmon in the oven with steamed vegetables on the side.

The amount of carbohydrates such as bread or potatoes or rice I add to my meals depends on the physical activity planned during the day.

10. SIMPLE DAILY RECIPES

CLASSIC SCRAMBLED EGGS
A Nutritious Breakfast Choice

Ingredients:
- 2 large eggs
- 2 tablespoons milk or cream (optional for creamier texture)
- Salt and pepper to taste
- 1 tablespoon butter or oil

Crack the eggs into a bowl. Add milk or cream (if using) and whisk until the mixture is smooth and slightly frothy.

Add a pinch of salt and pepper to the beaten eggs and mix well.

Place a non-stick skillet over medium-low heat. Add the butter or oil and let it melt and coat the pan.

Pour the egg mixture into the skillet. Let it sit for a few seconds without stirring. Gently stir the eggs with a spatula, pushing them from the edges to the center. Continue stirring until the eggs are just set but still slightly soft and creamy.

Remove the eggs from the heat and serve immediately.

TOASTED BREAKFAST DELIGHT
Egg, Cheese, and Ham

Ingredients:
- 2 slices of bread
- 1 large egg
- 1 slice of cheese (cheddar, Swiss, or your favorite)
- 1 slice of ham (or turkey, bacon, etc.)
- 1 tablespoon butter or margarine
- Salt and pepper to taste

Lightly butter one side of each slice of bread.

In a small pan over medium heat, crack the egg and cook until the white is set but the yolk is still soft. Season with salt and pepper.

Place the ham and cheese on the unbuttered side of one bread slice. Add the cooked egg on top.

Place the other slice of bread on top, buttered side facing out.

In a skillet over medium heat, cook the sandwich for about 2-3 minutes on each side, or until the bread is golden brown and the cheese is melted.

Remove from the skillet, cut in half if desired, and serve warm.

Enjoy your toasted breakfast delight!

HEALTHY TREAT
Yogurt with Honey and Walnut Topping

Ingredients:
- 1 cup plain Greek yogurt (or your favorite type)
- 2 tablespoons honey
- ¼ cup walnuts, chopped
- Optional: A pinch of cinnamon or fresh fruit for extra flavor

Place the yogurt in a bowl or cup.

Drizzle the honey over the yogurt evenly.

Sprinkle the chopped walnuts on top.

Add a pinch of cinnamon or fresh fruit like berries or banana slices if desired.

Enjoy immediately as a delicious and healthy snack or breakfast!

ITALIAN BEEF CARPACCIO
A Fresh and Flavorful Appetizer

Ingredients:
- 200g (7 oz) beef tenderloin or sirloin, very thinly sliced
- 2 tablespoons extra-virgin olive oil
- 1 tablespoon lemon juice
- A handful of arugula or mixed greens
- 2 tablespoons Parmesan cheese, shaved or grated
- Salt and freshly ground black pepper to taste
- Optional: Capers or thinly sliced red onion for garnish

Place the beef in the freezer for 15-20 minutes to firm up for easier slicing.

Slice the beef into very thin slices. Arrange them flat on a serving plate, slightly overlapping.

Drizzle the olive oil and lemon juice evenly over the beef slices.

Sprinkle with a pinch of salt and freshly ground black pepper.

Scatter the arugula or mixed greens over the beef.

Top with shaved or grated Parmesan cheese. Add optional capers or thinly sliced red onion if desired.

Serve immediately as a fresh and elegant appetizer.

FLAVORFUL BRESAOLA SALAD
Arugula, Cherry Tomatoes, and Cheese

Ingredients:
- 100g (3.5 oz) bresaola, thinly sliced
- 4 cups arugula (rocket) leaves
- 1 cup cherry tomatoes, halved
- 1/4 cup Parmesan cheese, shaved or grated
- 2 tablespoons extra-virgin olive oil
- 1 tablespoon lemon juice or balsamic vinegar
- Salt and freshly ground black pepper to taste

Place the arugula leaves on a serving plate or in a salad bowl.

Lay the thin slices of bresaola over the arugula.

Scatter the halved cherry tomatoes evenly over the salad.

Drizzle the olive oil and lemon juice or balsamic vinegar over the top.

Sprinkle with a pinch of salt and freshly ground black pepper.

Add the Parmesan cheese shavings or grated cheese on top.

Toss gently if desired and serve immediately.

Enjoy your refreshing and flavorful Bresaola Salad as a light lunch or appetizer!

DELICIOUS OMELETTE WITH CREAMY SAUCE

Ingredients:
- 3 large eggs
- 2 tablespoons milk or cream (optional for a fluffier omelette)
- Salt and pepper to taste
- 1 tablespoon butter or oil
- 2 tablespoons sour cream or crème fraîche
- Fresh chives, chopped

Crack the eggs into a bowl. Add the milk or cream (if using) and whisk until the mixture is smooth and slightly frothy.

Season with a pinch of salt and pepper.

Melt the butter or heat the oil in a non-stick skillet over medium heat until hot.

Pour the egg mixture into the skillet. Let it sit for a few seconds without stirring.

Gently lift the edges with a spatula, allowing the uncooked eggs to flow underneath. Continue until the omelette is mostly set but still slightly soft on top.

Once the eggs are mostly cooked, carefully fold the omelette in half or into thirds with the spatula.

Slide the omelette onto a plate. Spoon the sour cream or crème fraîche over the top.

Sprinkle the chopped fresh chives over the creamy sauce.

Serve immediately while the omelette is warm.

Enjoy your delicious omelette topped with a creamy sauce and fresh chives as a satisfying meal!

DELICIOUS GRILLED SALMON SERVED WITH STEAMED CARROTS AND BROCCOLI

Ingredients:
- 2 salmon fillets (about 150-200 grams each)
- 2 tablespoons olive oil
- 1 lemon, sliced (optional: use zest and juice for more flavor)
- Salt and freshly ground black pepper to taste
- 2 cups broccoli florets
- 2 large carrots, peeled and sliced into sticks

Preheat the grill to medium-high heat.

Brush both sides of the salmon fillets with olive oil and season with salt and pepper.

Optional: Squeeze a bit of lemon juice over the fillets for added flavor.

Place the salmon fillets skin-side down on the grill.

Grill for about 4-5 minutes per side, or until the salmon is opaque and flakes easily with a fork.

While the salmon is grilling, bring a pot of water to boil with a steaming basket placed above it.

Add the broccoli florets and carrot sticks to the steaming basket.

Cover and steam for about 5-7 minutes, or until the vegetables are tender but still slightly crisp.

Arrange the grilled salmon fillets on a plate.

Add the steamed carrots and broccoli alongside the salmon.

Optional: Garnish with lemon slices or a sprinkle of lemon zest for a fresh touch. Serve immediately and enjoy!

HEALTHY GRILLED CHICKEN SERVED WITH STEAMED BROCCOLI AND CARROTS

Ingredients:
- 2 boneless, skinless chicken breasts (about 150-200g each)
- 2 tablespoons olive oil
- 1 teaspoon dried herbs (such as oregano, thyme, or rosemary)
- Salt and freshly ground black pepper to taste
- 2 cups broccoli florets
- 2 large carrots, peeled and sliced into sticks
- Optional: Lemon wedges for serving

Preheat the grill to medium-high heat.

Brush both sides of the chicken breasts with olive oil. Season with salt, pepper, and dried herbs.

Place the chicken breasts on the grill. Cook for about 6-7 minutes per side, or until the chicken is cooked through and has nice grill marks. The internal temperature should reach 165°F (75°C).

While the chicken is grilling, bring a pot of water to boil with a steaming basket placed above it.

Add the broccoli florets and carrot sticks to the steaming basket.

Cover and steam for about 5-7 minutes, or until the vegetables are tender but still slightly crisp.

Arrange the grilled chicken breasts on a plate. Add the steamed broccoli and carrots alongside the chicken.

Optional: Squeeze lemon wedges over the chicken and vegetables for a fresh, zesty flavor.

Serve immediately while everything is hot and enjoy!

11. MY NUTRITION

My approach to nutrition is to adopt a balanced diet, which is crucial for overall health and provides the body with essential nutrients in the right proportions. A balanced diet has been shown to support effective diabetes management by improving glycemic control and reducing the risk of complications.

My nutrition plan is rich in protein because during these years, I have understood deeply the importance of protein intake. A study by Paddon-Jones and Leidy (2014) highlights that adequate protein consumption is essential for maintaining muscle mass, promoting recovery, and supporting metabolic health, which is particularly crucial as human beings age, but even more important for diabetes individuals. Protein is a crucial nutrient, for several important reasons mentioned in scientific studies, that I found to be true in myself.

- Blood Sugar Regulation: Protein-rich meals can help regulate blood sugar levels by slowing down the absorption of carbohydrates. I apply daily the strategy of combining carbohydrates with protein in order to flatten my glucose curve post meal.
- Muscle Health and Physical Activity: As I engage in regular physical activity, including endurance exercise, I need adequate protein for muscle repair and maintenance. During the weeks where my protein intake is not optimal I experience muscle pain and slower recovery.

MEAL	OPTION 1	OPTION 2	OPTION 3	OPTION 4
BREAKFAST 8:30 AM	200G 10% FAT QUARK 20G NUTS 50G BLUEBERRY 21P, 16C, 27F (400KCAL)	3 EGGS 30G 90% DARK CHOCOLATE 1 CAPPUCCINO 22P, 5C, 30F (380KCAL)	120G BREAD 30G CHICKEN SLICES 30G CHEESE 25P, 15C, 16F (315 KCAL)	200G YOGURT 30G NUTS 25P, 19C, 16F (335KCAL)
SNACK 10:30 AM	1 MANDARIN/ APPLE 16C (75KCAL)	2 KIWI 16C (90KCAL)	3 RICE CRACKERS 7P, 15C (150KCAL)	50G BREAD 15G CHICKEN 7P, 15C (105KCAL)
LUNCH 1:00 PM	80G CARPACCIO 15G PARMESAN 15 PINE NUTS 28P, 3C, 14F (250KCAL)	3 EGGS 20G CHEESE 20G HAM 200G VEGETABLES 29P, 0C, 21F (300KCAL)	80G TURKEY 120G BEANS 22P, 15C, 5F (265KCAL)	CAPRESE SALAD 100G BREAD 18P, 20C, 10F (270KCAL)
SNACK 5:00 PM	2 SLICE BROWN BREAD 30G CHEESE 30G CHICKEN 23P, 28C, 14F (320KCAL)	200ML YOGURT 2 TABLESPOON MUESLI 10G DRIED FRUIT 21P, 35C, 1F (330KCAL)	MELKUNIE PROTEIN DRINK 1 APPLE 21P, 32C, 4F (255KCAL)	MELKUNIE PROTEIN DRINK 10G DRIED FRUIT 21P, 32C, 4F (255KCAL)
DURING EXERCISE 18-20 PM	1 SPORT GEL 22C (90KCAL)	300ML ISOTONIC SPORT DRINK 20C (85KCAL)	1 SMALL BANANA 20C (85KCAL)	-
DINNER 9:00 PM	80G SALMON 200G VEGETABLES 1 TBS OIL 28P, 7C, 24F (320KCAL)	80G BREAD WITH REDUCED CARBS 3 EGGS 29P,15C,20F (370KCAL)	150G CHICKEN 50G MOZZARELLA 50G SPINACH 43P, 3C, 25F (410KCAL)	1 LOW CARB TORTILLA 60G BEEF 20G CHEESE 32P, 5C, 23F (375KCAL)

This table shows my nutrition plan for 2023-24 optimized with my nutritionist to get in shape for the race season. Explained the amount of C=Carbs, P=protein and F=fats.

- Weight Management: Protein contributes to satiety, helping myself feel full for a longer time. This played an important role in my weight management. I started consuming good quality protein as an afternoon or post dinner snack instead of carbohydrates or high fat options.
- Metabolism: Protein has a higher thermic effect compared to fats and carbohydrates, meaning the body burns more calories during digestion. This can be beneficial for overall metabolism.

The Recommended Dietary Allowance (RDA) for protein is 0.8 grams per kilogram of body weight for sedentary adults. However, athletes, including those with diabetes, may need higher amounts, typically ranging from 1.2 to 2.2 grams per kilogram of body weight.

Calculate Your Needs: Multiply your weight in kilograms by the recommended protein intake range (e.g., 1.2 to 2.2 grams). This gives you a range of protein intake in grams.

Example: If you weigh 70 kilograms and aim for 1.6 grams of protein per kilogram:

70 kg x 1.6 g/kg = 112 grams of protein per day
(within the range of 1.2 to 2.2 grams).

My nutrition plan is not only rich in protein and vegetables but also low in carbohydrates. When I initially reduced the amount of carbohydrates in my diet, I felt like something was missing. However, this feeling quickly dissipated when I began replacing carbohydrates with more protein and healthy fats. This shift helped me maintain energy levels and satiety, while also contributing to better blood sugar control and overall dietary satisfaction.

A study by Westman et al. (2007) supports this approach, demonstrating that low-carbohydrate diets can lead to improved glycemic control and increased satiety by enhancing protein and fat intake, making it a sustainable choice for managing diabetes.

After two weeks of adopting a low carbohydrate-based diet, my life positively changed. Adopting a high protein diet rich in vegetables stimulated the feeling of satiety. Surprisingly, during the day I was not feeling tired, hungry, or moody as they told me I would be feeling without carbs.

On the contrary, I felt better, less tired, less sleepy and experienced less brain fog during the day. The low carbohydrate diet had a direct impact on my glucose levels where I could observe a flat graph more often, without curves and spikes.

Why do a low carb and high protein diet work for me? Autoimmune diseases often come together, and in my case, diabetes T1 came with Hashimoto hypothyroidism. From literature I understood that a low carbohydrate diet can be beneficial for individuals with hypothyroidism for several reasons. Hypothyroidism often accompanies insulin resistance, and a low carb diet helps stabilize blood sugar levels and improve insulin sensitivity. By reducing carbohydrate intake, the body requires less insulin to manage blood glucose levels, which can be advantageous for individuals with hypothyroidism who might struggle with insulin resistance.

Hypothyroidism can lead to weight gain and difficulty in losing weight due to a slowed metabolism. Low carb diets promote weight loss by inducing a state of ketosis, where the body burns fat for fuel instead of carbohydrates. This helps manage weight more effectively, addressing a common challenge for those with hypothyroidism.

Inflammation is a common issue in hypothyroidism, especially in autoimmune thyroid conditions like Hashimoto's thyroiditis. Low carb diets tend to lower levels of pro-inflammatory markers in the body. Reducing carbohydrate intake, particularly refined sugars and processed foods, can decrease inflammation, potentially alleviating some symptoms associated with hypothyroidism.

A low carb diet improved my overall metabolic health by lowering triglycerides, increasing HDL (good) cholesterol, and improving LDL (bad) cholesterol particle size. These changes contributed to better heart health in my situation, which is important as hypothyroidism can be associated with an increased risk of cardiovascular disease.

Note: It's important for individuals with diabetes to work with healthcare professionals, including dietitians, to determine their specific protein needs based on their overall health, activity level, and diabetes management goals. Individualized recommendations can help optimize blood sugar control, support physical activity, and promote overall well-being.

12. DIABETES AND SPORT

In 2010, I was training with a swimming competition team in Turin. We trained four times a week in an indoor 25-meter pool. I loved swimming, especially with my friends, and I loved the feeling of being as strong as anyone else without diabetes. Yes, Gabriele and Tommaso, I was as strong as you guys! My swim trainer, Cesare never treated me differently because of diabetes but at the same time he made me feel understood and protected, giving me the possibility to get out of the pool if needed.

At the time, there were no CGM sensors, so to survive a 1 hour and 30-minute training session, I had to measure my blood glucose levels before, during, and after practice by pricking my finger and using a glucose meter. Different times, right?

Sometimes the training was so intense that the feeling of being tired could be confused with the feeling of hypoglycemia, or a real hypoglycemia event was difficult to detect because I was so focused on training. I brought my glucose monitoring kit to the edge of the pool so I could measure my glucose levels between reps without missing any training. This also allowed me to detect hypoglycemia and react with some sugar as soon as possible without walking all the way to the changing rooms.

One day, the coach came to me and told me my glucose kit was banned from the pool because some lap-swimming ladies had complained about seeing me prick my finger. From that day on, I was not allowed to have my glucose kit by the pool side anymore. Training and monitoring glucose levels is not only hard and challenging because it needs to be planned, monitored, and customized; it is also socially challenging! That experience made me even more expert at relying on my body sensations during sport. After all there is a positive side at the end of every story.

ENDURANCE TRAINING

Now, I am part of a triathlon club, Amsterdam Triathlon and Cycling (ATAC). I am surrounded by endurance athletes, and I wish to be as strong as them. I have noticed that both athletes with and without diabetes share many common nutritional principles, such as the need for proper fueling, hydration, and recovery. However, individuals with diabetes need to pay extra attention to managing blood sugar levels during training and competition, as this will influence the performance and the recovery. The focus for an athlete with diabetes is to balance the amount of carbs needed and optimize the timing of absorption.

During these three years as an endurance sport athlete and a scientist, I have gained unparalleled insights into the dynamic interplay between lifestyle factors and glucose management. My goal is not only to perform at my best but also to achieve a better body shape. Therefore, in the next pages, I will show my glucose levels during December and March 2022 while following a customized nutrition and exercise plan.

Keeping glucose levels stable is a difficult challenge, and understanding which foods to eat and in which order can be extremely beneficial. Adding training to the equation can make this challenge seem impossible! To handle glucose instability during physical activity, it's important to have a good starting glucose level before exercising, as it is normal for glucose to change rapidly during workouts. I make sure to start with a glucose level between 5.6 mmoL/L (100 mg/dL) and 5.6 mmoL/L (200 mg/dL) and have a fixed strategy in case of hyperglycemia or hypoglycemia.

As I consider myself an endurance athlete, I will dive into nutrition and glucose management for the three sports involved in triathlon: swimming, biking, and running. While many aspects of my diet align with general diabetes recommendations, there are specific considerations that require careful attention during sports.

First, I ensure that my caloric and energy needs are met, just like any other athlete. Maintaining this balance is essential for sustaining energy levels and supporting athletic endeavors. It's important to align carbohydrate intake with the energy expended during exercise to prevent hypoglycemia during workouts. Not only to avoid hypoglycemia but also to avoid muscle breakdown, it is good practice to start a workout with stable glucose levels and not on an empty stomach.

MY SPORTS STRATEGY

Engaging in endurance sports with type 1 diabetes requires meticulous planning and constant monitoring. Fortunately, continuous glucose monitors (CGMs) are a huge help, allowing us to check glucose levels instantly and anytime with a smartphone. I have used Freestyle Libre for a long time and now I am using the Dexcom G7. It easily connects with my Garmin watch and my Garmin bike computer, providing a significant benefit during training by allowing me to constantly monitor my glucose levels. Having my glucose data under control has made a big difference mentally as well as physically, alleviating the constant worry about low blood sugar.

The first step before every workout is to consider the type of exercise I am about to perform and its duration. I measure my glucose right before the activity and integrate if my glucose is below 100 mg/dL (5.6 mmoL/L). Usually, I integrate with slow releasing carbohydrates combined with protein if I anticipate a long aerobic activity that will decrease my glucose.

Even if I approach the exercise with stable glucose levels, I need to have a comprehensive understanding of my insulin requirements and carbohydrate intake to maintain stable blood sugar levels during exercise. This involves precise insulin dosing and the timing of carbohydrate consumption. After several attempts, I have identified what works for me nutrition-wise before starting an aerobic workout. I found it beneficial to consume small quantities of carbohydrates with different absorption speeds. For example, I consume an apple (15 grams fast-absorbing carbohydrates) and a slice of brown bread (15 grams of slow-absorbing carbohydrates).

While exercising, if I do not have my glucose monitor in front of me all the time, I check my glucose approximately every 30 minutes to assess if an adjustment is needed. After the workout, a key factor is consuming protein, as proteins are necessary to repair and build muscle tissue in response to the workout.

To standardize and optimize the nutrition process, regarding carbohydrate intake, I am working on an algorithm to calculate the carbohydrate intake needed for each person given the type, length, and intensity of workout they are about to face.

BEFORE TRAINING	DURING TRAINING	FTER TRAINING
considering exercise type, length, intensity. timing according to meals and glycemic trend	monitoring glycemia levels, especially if the activity exceeds 1 h	carbohydrates (cho) are necessary to reconstitute muscular and liver glycogen sources. liquids and sodium are necessary for rehydration
tools for cgm, equipped with increase and decrease glycemic indicators	consuming small quantities of cho with different absorption speeds	proteins are necessary to repair and assemble muscular tissue, in response to the workout
planning glycemic controls every 45 min–1 h	checking glycemia approximately every 30 min after training to establish the appropriate cho requirement	awareness of the risk of late hypoglycemia > up to 48 h later

The figure shows the glucose management advice before, during and after training.

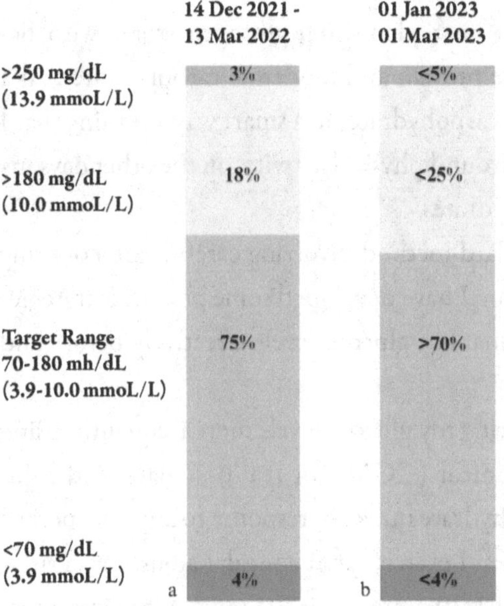

The figure shows the glucose graph summary using Freestyle Libre 2 for 90 days period from December 2021 till March 2022. Percentage on target between <70, 70 and 180, 181-240, >240. 75% of the time the glucose is on target with a balanced diet and daily exercise. Figure b shows the glucose graph summary using Dexcom G7 for 90 days during January 2023 and March 2023.

Balancing blood glucose levels during exercise can be a formidable task, particularly when the need to sustain optimal performance collides with the imperative of maintaining stable glucose. Depending on the type, length, and intensity of the training, I adjust my approach regarding insulin, nutrition, and target start and finish glucose value. I find it essential to fine-tune my insulin dosages and carbohydrate intake based on the demands of the exercise. For instance, I may reduce my basal insulin or take additional fast-acting carbohydrates before long and high-intensity workouts to prevent hypoglycemia. Most of the time, I try to perform endurance sports with a minimal active insulin deriving from my last bolus. This does not mean I exercise without insulin as I am using the pens, not an insulin pump, therefore I am never without basal insulin, meaning that there is always some basal active insulin in the body.

After exercise, I focus on replenishing glycogen stores with balanced meals that include protein and moderate carbohydrates. As I mention here, I consume carbohydrates in a smart way, meaning that I plan their consumption around physical activity, on the other days my diet is reduced in carbohydrates.

While I follow a standard method involving careful carb counting and insulin administration, I have developed some practical strategies or 'hacks' that help me manage glucose levels effectively before and after workouts.

These include monitoring my glucose levels more frequently, using a continuous glucose monitor (CGM) for real-time data, and adjusting my insulin or carbohydrate intake in response to any unexpected glucose fluctuations. When I exercise after a meal, I adjust my current insulin to carb ratio from 1:20 grams to 1:30 grams. Moreover, most of the time I reduce my basal insulin the day before if I am expecting an endurance effort the next day. This personalized approach allows me to maintain glucose stability and optimize my performance during various types of exercise.

- Avoid injecting insulin between two and two and a half hours before exercise.
- Make sure to have a banana or Gluc Up gel with me during the training.
- Combine fast absorption carbs with protein.
- Keep track of nutrition and glucose management.

Every day, I adjust my approach every single time towards sport and diabetes. Unfortunately, there is not a magical formula that tells me with exact precision what I should do but I started getting closer and closer to a personal strategy regarding insulin, nutrition, and target starting glucose levels to deal with exercises. For instance, Colberg et al. (2010) highlight the importance of adjusting insulin and carbohydrate intake to prevent hypoglycemia and maintain glucose stability during exercise.

Similarly, Riddell et al. (2017) discuss the benefits of tailoring insulin dosing and nutrition based on the specific demands of exercise to enhance performance and manage glucose levels effectively. I follow a standard method based not only on counting carbs and injecting insulin, but I also have some general hacks that I use before and after a workout. These include using real-time glucose monitoring to make immediate adjustments, taking fast-acting carbohydrates before high-intensity workouts, and ensuring balanced post-exercise meals to replenish glycogen stores and stabilize glucose levels.

One key strategy I use is to avoid having active (the bolus peak) insulin in the body, meaning not injecting insulin for two hours before exercise. In my experience, this helps prevent low glucose events during training. This approach frees you from the scary thoughts of hypoglycemia and allows you to enjoy the training to the fullest. Additionally, without peak active insulin, I could better understand how much the workout impacts my glucose levels.

Second, having a fixed integration strategy, such as using a banana for its fast absorption, is advantageous. It is safe during exercise and provides a consistent strategy for glucose management. This prevents random snacking and unplanned glucose spikes. Combining carbohydrates with different absorption rates helps keep glucose stable during aerobic workouts. The fast-absorbing glucose will enter the cells, creating small glucose spikes that will be flattened by the immediate effort, while the slow-absorbing carbs will keep the glucose curve flat.

Finally, keeping track of progress and failures is extremely important to understand what can be improved and what strategies should be maintained. Depending on the type of activity, I expect glucose to behave in specific ways, as shown in the figure below. While it is easy to understand why glucose decreases during a workout, it is less obvious why glucose increases. I will dive into different kinds of training to explain glucose predictability and the reasons behind these changes. At the same time, I will detail my behavior depending on the training I am about to perform.

EXERCISE TYPES AND GLUCOSE

Glucose trends vary depending on different work rates. The exercise could be aerobic, mixed, or anaerobic. There are many variables playing a role in the glucose trends, but the main ones are intensity and duration of the exercise, insulin active in the body, fitness level, nutrition, and initial glucose concentration.

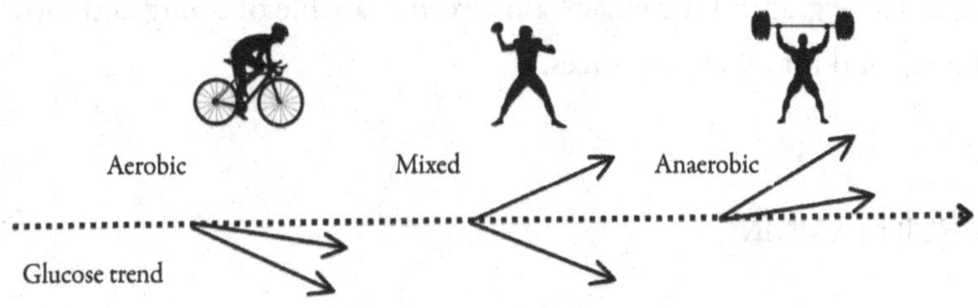

The figure shows the glucose trends during aerobic, mixed, and anaerobic workout.

LOW-IMPACT EXERCISES

Exercises such as yoga, pilates or stability training do not require specific nutritional preparation. I ensure my starting glucose is in range, not too low >3.9mmoL/L (>70 mg/dL) and not too high 13.9mmoL/L (<250 mg/dL). The security of having my glucose in the perfect rage allows me to stay fully focused and relaxed during the exercises. These types of exercises are beneficial for both the mind and body, as they reduce stress levels and body inflammation, consequently decreasing insulin resistance. A study by Melville et al. (2012) found that yoga and similar low-intensity exercises significantly reduce markers of inflammation and improve insulin sensitivity. I was pleasantly surprised to notice that this is indeed true. As my body relaxes, I experience a slow and gradual reduction in blood glucose in the hours following the exercise. My training plan includes a low impact session once or twice a week. Moreover, in case of body tiredness I change a hard session for a lower intensity session.

During these years I learnt not to ask too much from my body. I learnt to be grateful for what I am already capable of doing and most of all proud for all my sacrifices.

CARDIO TRAINING

Cardio training is an aerobic exercise that involves maintaining a moderate and steady heart rate. In order to sustain prolonged hours of cardio training I need to adopt a clear and defined strategy for my glucose management. I take this type of exercise very seriously, carefully planning the amount of insulin and carbohydrates I will need to sustain the activity. For example, according to a study by Colberg et al. (2010), proper carbohydrate intake before and during aerobic exercise is crucial for maintaining glucose levels and preventing hypoglycemia in individuals with diabetes. In my experience, depending on the training intensity, duration, fitness level, and the type of sport, glucose levels can drop at different rates.

To manage this effectively, I monitor my glucose levels closely before, during, and after the exercise, and I adjust my carbohydrate intake accordingly. My data collection over two years allowed me to perform a data analysis on my glucose values modulated by cardio exercise. The guideline I follow for my body, in order to avoid hypoglycemia, is to integrate 30 grams of fast carbohydrates every 40 minutes. This careful planning helps ensure that I have enough energy to sustain the workout without experiencing significant drops in blood glucose, thereby optimizing both my performance and safety during cardio training.

My bolus insulin dosage before exercise during a long cardio training session is reduced most of the time between 30 to 50% depending on the type of activity, duration and intensity. I would like to specify that as I use the insulin pens, I am never without insulin in the body as I have my 24 hours long lasting insulin always active.

STRENGTH TRAINING

Strength training is considered an anaerobic activity, and it is characterized by heart rate spikes. My training plan involved one or two sessions of strength every week. In my opinion, strength training is usually undervalued and not pursued correctly by women who prioritize cardio training, with the belief that it is more efficient to lose weight.

During my strength workout, I don't expect to experience low glucose events. If the strength training is a max effort training, the tendency is to experience a blood glucose increase. However, if strength training turns into endurance training with weight, glucose levels could drop steadily. Before strength training, I make sure my starting glucose is in range, not too low >3.9 mmoL/L (>70 mg/dL) and not too high <13.9 mmoL/L (<250 mg/dL), to perform heavy lifting safely and focus on technique exercises. Nutritionally, I ensure to eat the right amount of protein intake before and after the workout. Before, during and after exercise I check my glucose to avoid any hypoglycemia or hyperglycemia.

Below I will summarize the integration strategy I adopt if I am about to perform a mixed (aerobic and anaerobic) activity for 1 hour, like an endurance strength training session.

Under 65 mg/dL

- Assume 15g of simple and fast carbohydrates.
- Assume 20g of long-lasting carbohydrates.

Between 130-180 mg/dL: Assume 20g of long-lasting carbohydrates.

Above 250 mg/dL: Do not assume any food.

HYPERGLYCEMIA AND SPORT

At this point, I thought I had it under control. I had a nutrition strategy and an exercise strategy, but unexpectedly, during my training, I experienced an increase in blood glucose during anaerobic exercises and sometimes even during intense aerobic exercises.

During high-intensity aerobic and anaerobic exercise, glucose levels can increase due to the body's physiological response to stress. Stress hormones such as adrenaline and noradrenaline are released in response to the physical demands of intense exercise. These hormones stimulate the 'fight or flight' response, which increases heart rate, mobilizes energy stores, and promotes the release of glucose from the liver. This process helps provide a rapid source of energy necessary for sustained physical exertion.

According to research by Riddell and Perkins (2006), adrenaline and noradrenaline trigger the breakdown of glycogen, a stored form of glucose in the liver and muscles, converting it into glucose that enters the bloodstream. Additionally, cortisol, another stress hormone released by the adrenal glands, contributes to the increase in blood glucose by promoting gluconeogenesis—the formation of glucose from non-carbohydrate sources—and reducing glucose utilization in peripheral tissues. This combined hormonal action ensures that ample glucose is available to meet the heightened energy demands of the body during high-intensity exercise.

My current strategy to prevent hyperglycemia during high-intensity aerobic and anaerobic exercise is to adopt a low carb diet the day before the workout. Moreover, as I expect the glucose to rise sharply, I avoid eating carbohydrates before the start. Instead, I use protein and fat as a source of energy before the start.

Secondly, I avoid integrating in the first 30-40 minutes, even if the CGM suggests a slight drop in glucose levels during the first 40 minutes. After the first hour, I notice that the glucose tends to decrease and in that moment I start my integrations with long lasting carbohydrates.

Last but not least I do not reduce my insulin to carbs ratio, leaving it to the current level such as 1 unit of insulin per 20 grams, as I expect my glucose to increase.

Keeping the glucose in check while performing endurance high intensity aerobic activity, is extremely challenging without an insulin pump. In the near future I will be willing to discover the benefit of an insulin pump and overall diabetes management, now that the technology has made giant steps.

Lastly, as high-intensity exercise increases stress hormones, which can raise blood glucose levels. Unfortunately, the current trend of many diabetes instagram influencers is showing their training routine is often excessive, as it is not controlled by training coaches and healthcare specialists. The poorly managed high-intensity exercise may lead to prolonged stress hormone activity, potentially causing fatigue, impaired recovery, and increased risk of injury or illness. I try to incorporate stress management techniques like deep breathing, yoga, or meditation to help keep these levels in check.

13. BODY COMPOSITION

"Stop making excuses and start acting! The time for a change is now!" This is what I told myself at the beginning of 2022. I wanted to shape my body to feel better, feel lighter, run faster, swim longer, and improve my conditioning on the bike. I was tired of making excuses—"Not now," "I don't have time," "I'm too tired," "maybe tomorrow." I found my inner strength and took control of my own choices.

Many changes happened in my life in 2022. My parents got separated, I moved together with my boyfriend, I joined a triathlon club, I became active in volunteering, and all of these made me want to be the best version of myself. I wanted to feel good mentally and physically, getting rid of belly fat, improving my skin care, releasing muscular tension and starting a new home routine with stretching and yoga. Step by step I started taking control of my life, being patient and gentle with myself and with my diabetes. My mantra is "Diabetes is a rollercoaster, but it is your rollercoaster, you are the driver!". Every chapter I add some personal stories because I really want you to feel like you are in My Shoes, empathizing with emotions, struggles and also celebrating my victories. Moreover, I add my personal anecdotes as this book is a process of understanding my own body that took time and lots of steps were involved.

The nutrition strategy, the way of training, and the amount of insulin administered all play a role in my body composition. Body composition refers to the proportion of fat and nonfat mass in the body.

While individuals with diabetes may not necessarily have drastically different body compositions compared to those without diabetes, there are certain trends and associations that have been observed. It's important to note that individual variations exist, and not everyone with diabetes will have the same body composition. Here are some general observations supported by scientific evidence regarding body composition for people with diabetes:

- **Increased Fat Mass:** Research indicates that individuals with type 1 diabetes often have higher levels of body fat, especially visceral fat (fat stored around internal organs), compared to non-diabetic individuals. Therefore, elevated levels of visceral fat are associated with insulin resistance.

- **Changes in Fat Distribution:** People with diabetes may experience changes in fat distribution, with a tendency to accumulate fat around the abdominal region. This central or abdominal obesity is linked to insulin resistance and an increased risk of cardiovascular diseases. Studies have shown that the distribution of adipose tissue, particularly visceral fat, plays a role in the metabolic abnormalities seen in diabetes.

- **Lean Mass Alterations:** Studies suggest that individuals with diabetes may experience alterations in lean body mass. This can include a decrease in muscle mass, known as sarcopenia, which may contribute to difficulties in glycemic control. Loss of muscle mass can be associated with poor glucose metabolism and increased insulin resistance.

As I delved deeper into understanding my body, I recognized how profoundly nutrition, training, and insulin management influenced my body composition. Research shows that individuals with type 1 diabetes often carry increased visceral fat, a type linked to insulin resistance, as well as shifts in fat distribution and lean mass. These changes are critical to glycemic control and overall metabolic health. Learning this motivated me to explore my own data.

In 2022, I began monitoring my body weight with a scale and meticulously logging my nutrition and insulin intake. This marked a turning point—bringing greater awareness to my daily habits and how they influenced not just my body but my energy, performance, and glucose levels. This practice empowered me to make informed decisions and tailor my approach to fitness and diabetes management.

The journey to change isn't easy, but it is always worth it. Every choice, from the foods I eat to the insulin I administer, contributes to my ongoing process of becoming the healthiest version of myself. By sharing these stories and strategies, I hope to inspire others to take charge of their lives, stop making excuses, and embrace the opportunities for transformation that lie within.

MONITORING AND IMPROVING

On the 15th of June 2022, I started measuring my body composition using the In Body Balance machine available at my local gym in Amsterdam. This measurement provided me with important parameters for tracking my muscle mass, lean mass and fat mass. It was only a starting point, but it triggered my data driven personality to be consistent on my diet and training plan to have another measurement later in time. Consequently, I have tried to perfect my diet, train more efficiently, and give my body the right recovery time.

Being followed closely with healthcare specialists and personal trainers, my goal was to increase my overall health, perfecting my diet and training plan, with the secondary aim to also decrease the amount of insulin administered, as insulin is a hormone that stimulates adipose tissue accumulation. As I mentioned before, increased fat mass leads to insulin resistance, and insulin resistance requires more insulin to lower blood glucose levels. Moreover, high amounts of insulin can cause low glucose events, which increase the production of stress hormones. These stress hormones themselves contribute to an increase in adipose tissue, such as belly fat.

My advice is to try to keep glucose levels as stable as possible by adopting different strategies. Having more stable glucose levels will allow us to use less insulin and prevent the glucose rollercoaster.

Measuring weight, fat mass, and body fat max index (BMI) is important because these parameters could influence insulin sensitivity. Excess body fat, especially visceral fat, can reduce insulin sensitivity, making it harder to manage blood glucose levels. Maintaining a healthy BMI and lower fat mass can enhance insulin effectiveness.

Moreover, maintaining a good weight and BMI could help reaching a good blood glucose control as proper BMI and lower fat mass can lead to more stable blood glucose levels, reducing the risk of both hyperglycemia and hypoglycemia.

In summary, keeping BMI and fat mass under control is crucial for individuals with Type 1 diabetes to enhance insulin sensitivity, reduce cardiovascular risks, maintain stable blood glucose levels, prevent complications, and optimize physical performance.

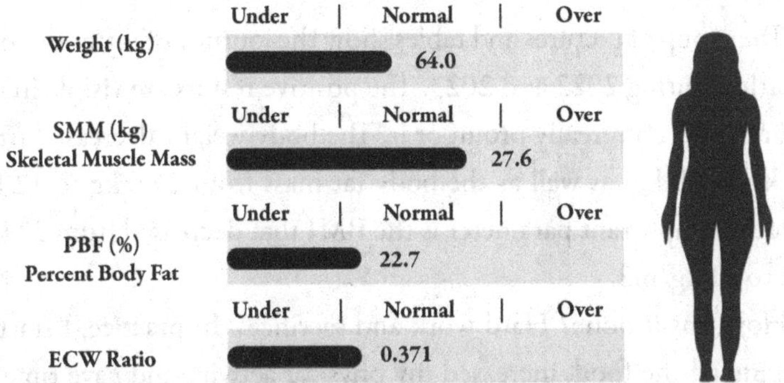

The figure shows my result of the body measurement for weight, Skeletal Muscle Mass (SMM), Percent Body Fat (PBF), ECW Ratio.

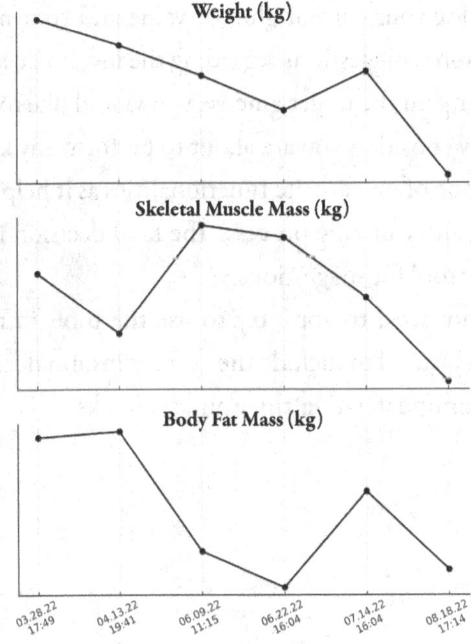

Tracking body composition trends in time: BMI, body fat, lean mass, and ECW Ratio.

The group of pictures and tables show the journey of my body composition during 2022 and 2023. The positive results are visible in the figures, and I am really proud of it. The body weight decreased from 64 kg to 60 kg, as well as the body fat mass from 14.5 kg to 12 kg. Another important parameter is the BMI that decreased from 22 kg/m2 to 21 kg/m2.

How was it done? Hard work and sacrifices. In practice, I started logging all the food, increased my physical activity and gave time to my body to sleep and recover.

Logging the food can be pretty overwhelming, one amazing app I consider beneficial is Dally. Dally is a diabetes user-friendly app that allows you to log your current glucose value and your nutrition. The app gives you some suggestions regarding the insulin doses you should inject depending on the target glucose you would like to achieve after the meal. Dally considers you are about to perform any kind of exercise, and this is one of my favorite functionalities as it helps me with decision making and thinking process. The final decision is always ours but it is a great tool for suggestions.

If you are not used to apps, try to use the tools in the following table. This can be used to include the current insulin dosage plan with placeholders for updates after three and six weeks.

MEAL	UNITS	INSULIN TYPE	INSULIN UNITS AFTER 3 WEEKS	INSULIN UNITS AFTER 6 WEEKS
BREAKFAST				
LUNCH				
SNACK				
DINNER				
SNACK				

This table allows insulin dosage tracking over time. The table shows the daily insulin unit, insulin type, date.

14. INFLUENCE OF HORMONES

I want to picture myself as a disciplined endurance athlete with type 1 diabetes, preparing for the Amsterdam Half Marathon. During training sessions, I have developed a precise understanding of how my body responds to exercise, and I have fine-tuned my insulin dosages, carbohydrate intake, and hydration strategies accordingly.

For the half marathon, I prepared by doing long runs on weekends and short interval runs during the week. Amsterdam is beautiful, full of parks where many runners meet and run together. Vondelpark is my fixed running trail where I could relax mentally and focus on my breathing. When I go running, I always carry my running belt with my phone, sugar, gels, and sometimes a glucose machine in case my CGM fails. During the training sessions, I typically maintained stable blood glucose levels by meticulously balancing insulin and carbohydrate intake to ensure optimal performance. My goal is to to start running with stable glucose levels, making sure to ingest some long-acting carbohydrates around 30 minutes before starting, as I expect a long and steady effort.

However, when the day of a major competition arrives, the scenario changes. Here we are at my Half Marathon. Logically, I expected to experience low blood sugar during the competition, so I prepared with an insane number of gels and protein bars. Surprisingly, I experienced high glucose levels while performing three hours of aerobic activity. In the last 5 km of the race, my glucose levels were too high, and I started experiencing fatigue. I decided to inject one unit of insulin that I carried with me into my running belt. Despite this unexpected situation, I managed to cross the finish line with joy and satisfaction.

This situation presents a delicate balancing act, where I had to continuously monitor my blood glucose levels and make informed decisions about insulin administration and carbohydrate intake during the race to mitigate the impact of elevated glucose levels. The stress of competition adds a layer of complexity to diabetes management, necessitating adaptability and meticulous planning to ensure a successful and safe endurance sport experience.

Ensuring an optimized nutrition strategy is important to prevent both low and high glucose events. Elevated glucose levels can potentially lead to the formation of lactic acid, which, in turn, can cause feelings of weariness. While concrete scientific evidence about the detrimental effects of high glucose during short-term exercise remains inconclusive, personal experiences often tell a vivid story. Individuals like me have reported difficulties in breathing and muscle soreness when glucose levels soar above 250 mg/dL (13.9 mmoL/L).

Performing physical activity with elevated glucose isn't an outright contraindication, but it can present a hurdle to achieving one's full potential. When glucose levels are too high, the body may struggle to perform at its peak, affecting an athlete's ability to give 100%. This performance compromise is why meticulous glucose management is a critical facet of the journey.

When I arrived home, I started reading scientific articles about it and discovered that competition stress in individuals with type 1 diabetes often leads to a noticeable elevation in blood glucose levels compared to the relatively stable levels observed during a training exercise session at the same intensity.

THE IMPACT OF COMPETITION

This phenomenon is primarily attributed to the distinct glucose trends that become evident in the period leading up to the competition. During this pre-competition phase, I often experience anticipatory stress, which significantly influences my blood glucose levels. To illustrate the magnitude of this effect, it's insightful to reference the experience of T1D Olympic swimmer Gary Hall, Jr., who observed a remarkable spike in his blood glucose levels during a 50-meter race. Hall reported that his blood glucose levels could surge from 5.6 mmoL/L (100 mg/dL) to 16 mmoL/L (300 mg/dL) in just 21 seconds.

During high-intensity physical activity, such as a competitive race, the body engages in heightened hepatic glycogenolysis, the process of breaking down glycogen stored in the liver to release glucose into the bloodstream. These delicate physiological interactions are the unique challenges I faced during competitions. When I decided to engage in competitive sports, this mechanism was new to me. In fact, the graphs of my first competitions are a rollercoaster of emotions and sugar peaks. After these years, I have gained a comprehensive understanding of these processes and developed effective strategies for managing blood glucose during such high-pressure events.

To avoid high glucose levels during exercise, some individuals may consider increasing their insulin dosage. However, this too is a balancing act and needs to be executed perfectly, with the advise of healthcare specialists.

THE POST-WORKOUT

I love going on long bike rides, but they sometimes bring a tough opponent: glucose spikes afterwards. Have you ever experienced that after a workout?

It's like my body reacts inducing hyperglycemia as soon as it is relaxed. One day, after about 3 hours riding my bike, my blood sugar levels suddenly started to rise. Confused regarding what was going on, I kept pushing on the bike till finally I arrived home. To prevent severe hyperglycemia, I corrected it with insulin but unexpectedly the glucose spikes up even more without responding to insulin as it is used to. Let me tell you the full story now.

It was a usual cloudy and windy Saturday. Saturday is the day where I usually go on bike rides, starting in the morning, from 10:00 am. Repeatedly, what I have observed is that the glucose spiked after the workout, around midday. It felt like my body, tired from all the riding, decided to ignore the insulin I was injecting. Tired and hungry from the bike rides, the only thing I wanted to do when home was to start eating. Unfortunately, instead I needed to control my blood sugar and delay the eating time.

My glucose levels stubbornly stayed high for hours. In response, I had to keep a close eye on my blood sugar and inject myself with little insulin every couple of hours to try to bring the glucose level down.

But here's the tricky part, as my stress level dropped when home, my body consequently started to relax, and I noticed that my blood sugar would suddenly drop. This sudden drop made me feel dizzy, with a racing heart, just plain uncomfortable. Dealing with this situation shows how important it is for people like me with type 1 diabetes who enjoy long workouts, to find the right balance, test different nutrition protocols and be careful with post workout hyperglycemia. I learned that It's not just about knowing my body but also being flexible and adjusting your plan to perform well and stay healthy.

Why was this after exercise spike happening? I began analyzing my behavior before and during exercise.

Before exercising, I reduce my insulin dosage to prevent hypoglycemia during the workout. While this is a proactive measure, it can result in a shortage of active insulin in the body post-exercise, causing glucose levels to rise. Another factor is delayed carbohydrate absorption. When I consume carbohydrates during exercise, the body's focus shifts towards supplying energy to the working muscles. As a result, the absorption and utilization of carbohydrates can be temporarily delayed. The carbohydrates I consume might not have an immediate impact on blood sugar levels during physical activity, as they are stored in the liver and muscles as glycogen, ready to be released when needed.

Diabetes management would be much easier without stress, sicknesses, menstrual cycle and competitive sport. Everything was so much smoother before physical activity became part of the game. I not only noticed glucose spikes during high-intensity activities, such as competitions, but also after intense workouts or competitions. While achieving peak performance during training or competition is the goal, experiencing a spike in blood glucose levels after exercise can be as bothersome as a toothache. So, what's behind this often-unwelcome post-workout increase in blood sugar levels?

I have experienced sugar peaks after workouts and decided to investigate the science behind it. Several factors contribute to the rise in blood sugars after exercise, and understanding these intricacies is essential for effective diabetes management. As I try to reduce active insulin during my workout, one significant contributor is the insufficient presence of active insulin in the body post-exercise. This deficiency often occurs when insulin infusion rates are intentionally reduced (as in my case) or when a smaller insulin dose is administered before or during the workout. As a result, the body has limited insulin available to process the carbohydrates consumed.

Additionally, the carbohydrates I consume during exercise may exhibit a delayed release into the bloodstream. During physical activity, the body prioritizes the delivery of energy to the working muscles, which can temporarily impede the normal absorption and utilization of carbohydrates. Consequently, these carbohydrates might be released into the bloodstream after the exercise has concluded.

When this release coincides with a state of reduced insulin availability, it can lead to a swift and noticeable surge in blood sugar levels. This effect becomes even more pronounced if you continue to eat or drink carbohydrates after your exercise, compounding the post-workout glucose increase.

It's crucial to recognize that various exercise intensities, durations, and individual responses can influence the degree of post-workout blood sugar fluctuations. Moreover, the timing of your meal or snack before exercise, as well as the type and quantity of carbohydrates consumed during exercise, plays a pivotal role in determining the magnitude of the post-exercise blood sugar rise.

My personal stories I share are rich in insight and mistakes to which I have learned how to achieve a delicate balance between insulin dosing, carbohydrate intake, and the timing of exercise.

LATE CARBOHYDRATE RELEASE

During my long bike rides or long run it is needed to have a nutrition strategy in place, in order to sustain such a prolonged effort avoiding hypoglycemia. Usually, I keep integrating every 30-40 minutes with gels. After having tried different gel brands, The Gluc Up became my favourite as it is composed of 15 grams of glucose, which raises my glucose very fast, without other long carbohydrates inside.

Most of the glucose contained in the gels gets absorbed straight away but not all of it. When will these remaining carbohydrates contained in most of the gels get released? Post-exercise!

I have noticed that once I have completed my workout, my body starts to relax to initiate the recovery. During this recovery phase, the carbohydrates that were stored as glycogen during exercise can be released into the bloodstream. This can lead to an increase in blood sugar levels, particularly if there's limited active insulin available to facilitate the uptake of this glucose by the cells.

Understanding this science is crucial for me as a diabetic athlete. It empowers me to make informed decisions about insulin dosing, carbohydrate intake, and the timing of exercise. Achieving a harmonious balance between these factors is key to effectively managing blood sugar levels during and after physical activity. I am not going to lie, saying it is easy, on the contrary it is a huge challenge, but not impossible to achieve.

Thanks to years of practice and data collection I have figured out the exact amount of carbohydrates needed for myself to successfully complete training without experiencing low glucose events and avoiding severe hyperglycemia due to late carbohydrates release. Therefore,

I can roughly predict how much my glucose will drop during different kinds of exercises and intensities, which means optimizing nutrition and insulin administration. To do so, I have conducted various tests, monitoring my glucose levels before and after exercise keeping track of the amount of carbohydrates eaten.

15. GLUCOSE VARIABILITY

Despite maintaining a balanced and controlled diet, my glucose levels could fluctuate due to various factors, such as sickness, stress, and the menstrual cycle. Despite being very grateful for what I have in my life, I am subject to stress. For me happiness does not mean to have everything I want, happiness means to be happy with what I have. Luckily, the emotional and financial support from my parents was never lacking, which allowed me to start a new life and career in Amsterdam.

Despite having a strong and positive mindset, my glucose values are heavily affected by stress, sickness and menstrual cycle hormones. Stress is a complicated physical reaction that is closely connected to the release of cortisol and can be a major challenge for people with type 1 diabetes. I have noticed that when I am stressed because of work, relationships, or personal problems, hormones like cortisol can lead to changes in blood sugar levels and require more insulin to regulate.

Cortisol, the main stress hormone, plays a key role in releasing glucose from the liver, making it harder for tissues to absorb glucose, and causing insulin resistance. Additionally, when the sympathetic nervous system is activated due to stress, it releases epinephrine and norepinephrine, which raise blood sugar levels by increasing glucose production in the liver. Stress, whether ongoing or sudden, disrupts the balance between insulin and glucose, resulting in unpredictable blood sugar levels and a higher risk of high blood sugar.

When dealing with high blood sugar levels before exercise, it is important to be cautious. While it may seem logical to take extra insulin to lower blood sugar, the situation may, however, become more complex when I am getting ready to do a challenging 10 km run or a tough 40 km bike ride. Even though I am experiencing lower insulin sensitivity and higher blood sugar, because of stress, the insulin injected starts working better, and faster, leading to a significant drop in my blood sugar levels while I am exercising. This is because the injected insulin starts to work more effectively, leading to a sudden decrease in blood sugar during exercise.

In addition, dealing with the menstrual cycle makes things more complicated. Before and during my period, my blood sugar is more likely to rise and maintain higher values. The hormonal changes during this time can make my body less responsive to insulin, leading to higher and fluctuating blood sugar levels. It's important to have a plan to manage these hormonal effects. I try to stabilize my blood sugar by not only taking the right amount of insulin but also maintaining a healthy lifestyle.

Factors like stress, hormones, and illness can cause insulin resistance in my body, requiring me to increase the amount of insulin I usually need. How can I get my blood sugar levels back to normal? Unfortunately, it takes time for my body to adjust to the new stress and return to normal levels. I have understood it is fundamental to treat my body with love and compassion. Here are some strategies that help me manage my glucose levels during stressful times:

- Increase the insulin doses carefully and progressively (Always with the help of health care advice).
- Avoid sweets (e.g chocolate) and processed food.

- Move extra 15 minutes every day.
- Practice Yoga and meditation.

INFECTIONS

In response to infection, the body releases stress hormones like cortisol and adrenaline. These hormones increase glucose production in the liver and decrease the effectiveness of insulin, leading to higher blood glucose levels. Moreover, infection-induced inflammation can make the body's cells less responsive to insulin, further exacerbating hyperglycemia.

Depending on the types and seriousness of infections the blood sugar level is impacted differently.

Minor infections typically cause a temporary increase in blood glucose levels. Proper management and recovery usually return levels to normal within a few days. On the contrary, flu or gastroenteritis can cause more significant and prolonged hyperglycemia due to higher stress hormone levels, more pronounced inflammation, and potential dehydration. Blood glucose levels may remain elevated for a week or more, depending on the infection's severity and the individual's response.

In summary, viral and bacterial infections can significantly impact blood glucose levels in individuals with Type 1 diabetes, with the severity and duration of this impact varying based on the infection's seriousness. Effective management strategies, including frequent monitoring, adjusting insulin dosage, staying hydrated, and seeking medical attention, are crucial to mitigate these effects.

The pictures have the aim to show the impact of sicknesses on the blood glucose. Comparing the graphs it is visible how the glucose levels stay elevated during a 24 hour period during a sick week, compared to glucose levels returning to normal in a range over 24 hours in a normal week.

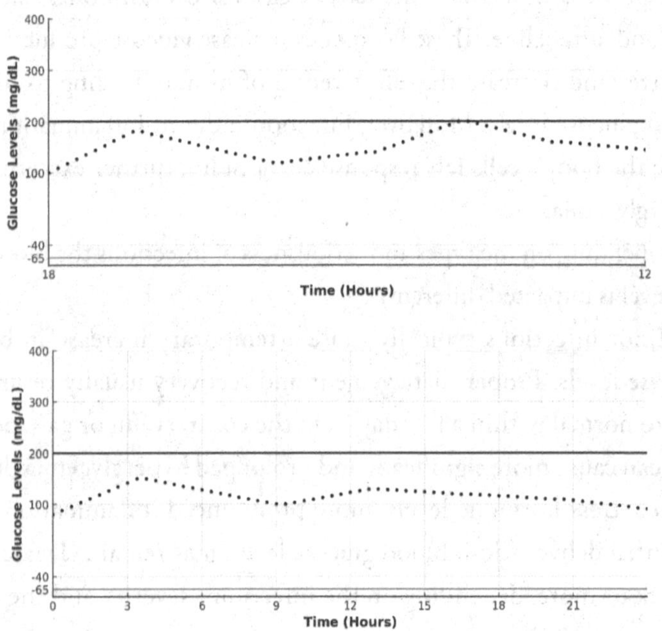

The figure is Dexcom G7 24-hour blood glucose monitoring extract comparison between a sick week and a healthy week. Observable glucose is mostly high during the sick week (upper figure).

STRESS

Stress has a huge and often underestimated impact on diabetes management. The stress-induced insulin resistance is a substantial factor influencing glucose spikes. Life events, such as university exams, pressure to deliver at work, family sicknesses are not immune to the ramifications of heightened stress, leading to undesirable fluctuations in blood sugar levels. This stress-induced insulin resistance can manifest after distressing incidents or during the menstrual period, adding yet another layer of complexity to diabetes management. With the assumption that my lifestyle does not change, following a standard diet and daily exercises, these two graphs represent morning with a stressful meeting at work and a relaxed morning.

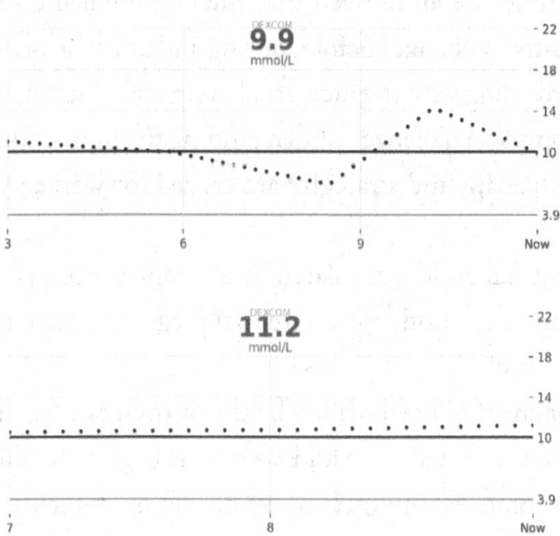

The figure shows the impact of stress on blood glucose levels: stressful vs. regular meeting. The upper figure a shows the hyperglycemia consequently a stressful meeting while the lower shows my glucose jumping for a not stressful meeting.

MENSTRUAL CYCLE

Women are not small man, is the Ted talk title given by Stacy Sims. All my life, I trained the very same way as the men were doing, I was suggested a nutrition strategy same as the men, without taking into account a huge difference between the two sexes: The menstrual cycle. This impacts female health and lifestyle in a huge way. Finally, in 2023, we started talking more about it, in the Amsterdam Triathlon and Cycling club. The Menstrual cycle not only influences the way a female athlete should train but also influences the performance, the lifestyle that has to be modified week by week.

In this book, we are talking not only about female athletes, but athletes with diabetes. What is the impact on blood sugar? For the women reading, we all noticed that the blood glucose stability and insulin sensitivity changes before, during and after the period.

In short, dealing with the menstrual cycle, stress, and managing diabetes is a complex challenge. Understanding the body's functions and being able to adapt and strategize are crucial for women with type 1 diabetes.

The menstrual cycle is regulated by a complex interplay of hormones that prepare the body for a potential pregnancy each month. These hormones include:

- **Estrogen:** Produced mainly by the ovaries, estrogen helps regulate the menstrual cycle and is responsible for the thickening of the endometrial lining. It peaks during the follicular phase and again just before ovulation.
- **Progesterone:** Produced by the corpus luteum in the ovaries after ovulation, progesterone stabilizes the endometrial lining,

making it suitable for implantation of a fertilized egg. If pregnancy does not occur, progesterone levels fall, leading to menstruation.

- **Follicle-Stimulating Hormone (FSH):** Produced by the pituitary gland, FSH stimulates the growth of ovarian follicles, each containing an egg, during the first half of the cycle.
- **Luteinizing Hormone (LH):** Also produced by the pituitary gland, LH triggers ovulation (the release of a mature egg from the ovary) and the formation of the corpus luteum.
- **Gonadotropin-Releasing Hormone (GnRH):** Secreted by the hypothalamus, GnRH stimulates the pituitary gland to release FSH and LH.

This technical introduction, might seem boring but that helped me understanding the root cause of my glucose fluctuation. Following I will deep dive into the different menstrual cycle phases: Follicular and Luteal.

Estrogen tends to improve insulin sensitivity, which can help lower blood glucose levels, while Progesterone generally causes insulin resistance, leading to higher blood glucose levels. This hormone's effect is more pronounced in the second half of the menstrual cycle (the luteal phase).

- Follicular Phase (Day 1 to 14): During this time the Estrogen levels rise, which can improve insulin sensitivity and may result in lower blood glucose levels. According to literature, women with diabetes may find it easier to manage their blood sugar during this phase. My experience confirms this finding, as well as I demonstrate in the pictures.

- Ovulation (Around Day 14): This is a critical phase as a surge in LH and FSH occurs, and estrogen is at its peak. The insulin sensitivity is usually at its highest.
- Luteal Phase (Day 15 to 28): In the second part of the menstrual cycle phases, the progesterone levels rise, leading to increased insulin resistance. According to literature, women may experience higher blood glucose levels and may need to adjust their insulin or medication dosages. During these years of self-observation I found the same pattern on my glucose levels.
- Menstruation (Day 1 to 5 of the next cycle): During the menstruation phase, the hormone levels drop, and insulin sensitivity may increase again. Blood glucose levels may stabilize or decrease.

What I have observed on my glucose levels, over the period of more than a year, is exactly what literature has proved. I have been looking, comparing and analyzing my data from Dexcom G7, with the aim to first understand why my glucose level was fluctuating in such unpredictable ways.

The conclusion of my observation is a stabilization of the glucose levels during the menstruation day 1-5. My glucose is more prone to hypoglycemia events during the so-called, bleeding days. During the following follicular phase, the glucose management is easier, as the insulin sensitivity increases. In this period of time, I feel more energized, and my body is more stress resistant.

On the contrary during the luteal phase, my glucose demonstrated to me more prone to hyperglycemia. The same amount of insulin would not have the same effects in lowering the blood glucose, resulting in an evident lower insulin sensitivity.

I ran an experiment for half a year where I wanted to demonstrate with data that the menstrual cycle has a profound impact in the glucose management for women. This factor is something that I have never taken into account but should be the baseline for the insulin management.

My experiment had some fixed parameters such as fixed insulin doses, fixed nutrition and fixed training schedule. In order to make sure to have as little interference as possible, I avoided parties and drinking nights, yes!

The conditions have been standardized for the entire experiment, recording and tracking my data with continuous glucose monitoring.

The conclusion is that during the first two weeks (Follicular Phase), my glucose levels were 85% of the time in range, showing an optimal insulin sensitivity. In the second week, I experienced the same easy feeling in managing my glucose although I could see more glucose variability towards the low and the high points. Progressively during the third and fourth week (Luteal Phase) the same units of insulin started having less effect for the same amount of carbohydrates, causing higher blood sugar values. As a result, I was in range 70% of the time compared to the 85% of the time of the Follicular phase.

As a result, female hormones play an important role in the glucose management but also on the overall energy levels and stress level. All these parts are connected with each other and influence the glucose variability and insulin resistance. The picture that represents the menstrual cycle stress, divided in two phases, follicular and luteal, shows the stress resistance level that an average woman could handle through the different phases of the menstrual cycle. Women are more stress resistant in the two weeks of the follicular phase and the beginning of the first part of the Luteal phase.

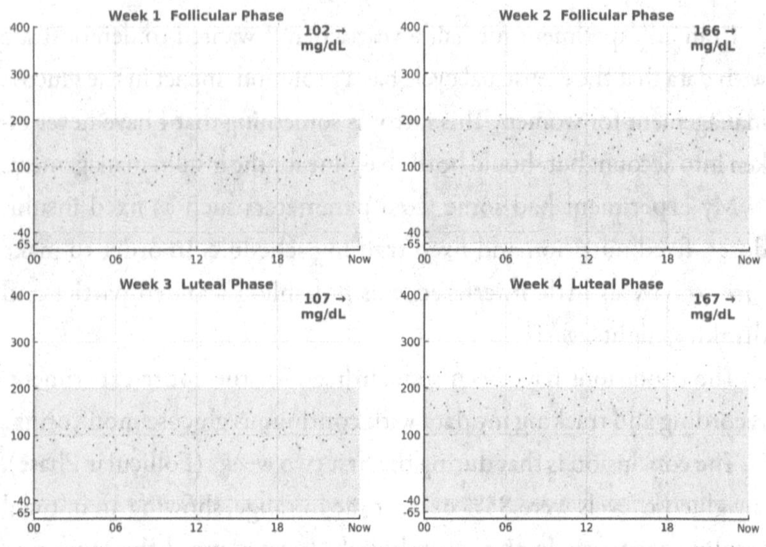

The table represents how the menstrual cycle hormones influence the glucose levels during four weeks.

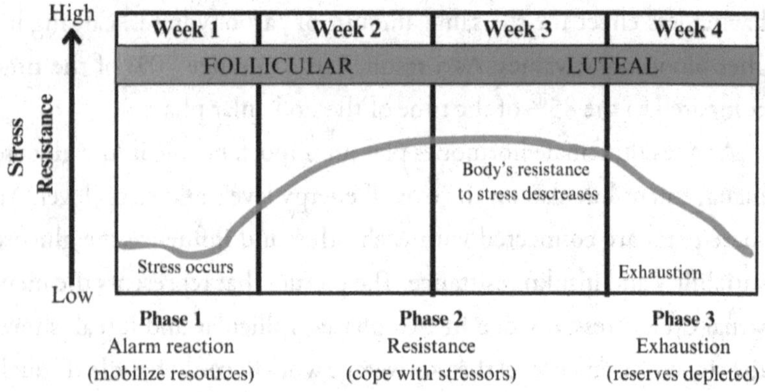

The table represents the stress resistance level that an average woman has through the different phases of the menstrual cycle. Women are more stress resistant in the two weeks of the follicular phase and the beginning of the first part of the luteal phase.

The menstrual cycle significantly influences glucose levels, energy levels, and stress resistance due to hormonal fluctuations, which women with diabetes should carefully consider when managing their health and shaping their training routines. During the follicular phase, the body is generally more stress-resistant, and insulin sensitivity tends to be higher, making this phase an optimal time for higher-intensity training sessions. Blood glucose levels are typically more stable, and energy levels are consistent, allowing for better performance and recovery.

As women transition into the luteal phase, hormonal changes, including increased progesterone levels, can reduce insulin sensitivity, leading to higher glucose variability and potentially decreased energy levels. This phase may require adjustments in insulin dosing and a focus on moderate-intensity activities, emphasizing endurance or recovery-based training. Additionally, the second half of the luteal phase may bring increased stress sensitivity and fatigue, so incorporating rest days and mindfulness practices can be beneficial.

Understanding these physiological variations empowers women to tailor their training plans to their cycle phases, optimizing performance while minimizing the risk of glucose instability. This approach not only enhances athletic outcomes but also supports overall well-being, providing a holistic strategy for managing diabetes and maximizing physical and mental resilience throughout the cycle.

16. TRIATHLON TRAINING

Triathlon is more than a hobby for me, it became a safe space that allows me to feel good, get rid of stress and anxieties. Triathlon is the place where I found life long lasting friendships and discovered my truly inner strength. Triathlon is a great sport because activities like swimming, biking, and running are excellent cardiovascular exercises. They help improve circulation, enhance heart health, and manage blood pressure—crucial factors for individuals with diabetes to prevent complications.

Regular swimming, biking, or running contributed to weight control and helped me maintain a healthy body mass index (BMI), a key aspect in managing diabetes, as excess weight can exacerbate insulin resistance. Over time, I noticed that physical activity increases insulin sensitivity, allowing my body to utilize glucose more efficiently. This can aid in stabilizing blood sugar levels, a fundamental aspect of diabetes management.

I always loved training, the feeling of being invincible at the end of a hard one. The satisfaction in my eyes and in my training buddies eyes which releases endorphins from every pore.

THE BENEFITS OF SWIMMING

During a rainy Sunday in Amsterdam in 2022, I decided to go swimming in a 50 meters pool that I discovered a couple of weeks earlier. I was very excited as I had never swum before in an Olympic distance pool! The pool was and it still is, beautiful, spacious, clean, and had big windows looking towards the lake that allowed me to look outside and imagine myself swimming in a crystal-clear sea. As usual, I got changed and checked my glucose through my phone at the beginning of the session. I left all my belongings in the locker apart from my phone, which I put in a waterproof case, and I made sure to carry it with me by the poolside. The reason why I carry my phone with me is to prevent sensor errors caused by lost connections that might require the need to replace the sensor. On a second note, It allows me to check my glucose during training if needed.

I jumped into the water and a feeling of happiness passed through my body. Tommaso, my Italian swimming friend, sent me a workout to follow for that day, arranged by our swim instructor back in Turin. The plan consists of training 100 meters and 50 meters freestyle repetitions at high intensity pace. I remember I was trying to keep up with a couple of fast swimmers in my lane. During a recovery break, one of the swimmers asked me if I liked the Supersapiens on my arm and if it was working well. I found out later that Supersapiens is an arm glucose monitor for triathletes, looking and functioning exactly in the same way as freestyle libre, or Dexcom G7 for people with diabetes. The only difference is that it is more expensive and not covered by insurance, but allows people without diabetes to monitor their blood glucose. I told them I had no idea what they were talking about, but my arm scanner was functioning very well because I have type 1 diabetes.

I explained that the patch was a necessity for me because of my chronic condition and unfortunately, I was not a triathlete. His face was surprised, and he was disappointed with my lack of feedback about

Supersapiens, but he encouraged me to join the Amsterdam triathlon club, ATAC. Excited, I went home and subscribed! Nicky and Jose, the guys in the pool, soon would not only become my friends, but Jose also my triathlon coach.

That day I will remember it forever as was the start of a beautiful journey but also the first time someone saw my arm scanner and thought I was an athlete, not someone sick. There are more and more stories about what people thought and told me regarding my arm scanner, and perhaps this could be a book on its own; nicotine patch, portable WIFI, inflatable doll...

Coming back to swimming; This is my favorite sport as I feel relaxed and light-weight in the water while gaining the cardiovascular and muscular benefits of a full-body activity. Swimming is a low-impact exercise that is gentle on the joints, making it suitable for individuals with diabetes, like me, who may experience joint issues. In the past, I suffered from a slipped disk in my lower back 4-5L, and I have an ongoing knee problem with my meniscus. Swimming allows me to consistently exercise without causing additional stress on my body.

My swimming training with ATAC takes place two or three times a week. I train at different times of the day: early morning from 7:00 am to 8:00 am, lunchtime from 13:00 pm to 15:00 pm, or evening from 19:00 pm to 20:00 pm.

Below is an example of swim training sessions. My nutrition for the swimming session most of the time includes 30 grams of fast acting carbohydrates, such as an apple, and 20 grams of slow acting carbohydrates, such as a slice of brown bread. Despite the high-intensity training, the graph shows that my glucose levels manage to remain in range during the hour, avoiding hypoglycemia or hyperglycemia after the workout.

Swimming training can vary in duration and intensity (tables on the next page), but my nutrition strategy remains the same and consistent every time. From my experience, this consistency is key to reducing unexpected hypoglycemic or hyperglycemic events during training and allows me to focus on performance.

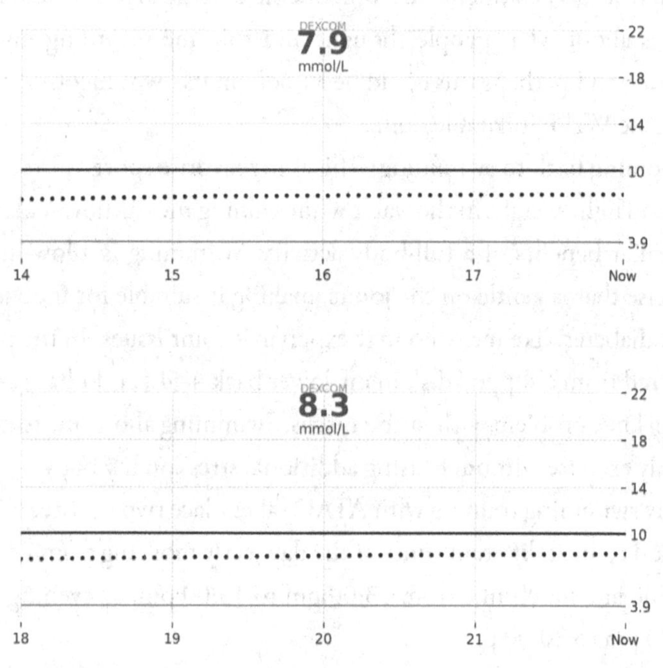

The graphs show the glucose values recorded with Dexcom G7 during swimming training.

TIME	STAGE	TYPE	Distance (m)
07:00-07:15	WARM UP	OWN CHOICE	3X100
07:15-07:30	TECHNIQUE	FREESTYLE	4X150
07:30-07:45	TECHNIQUE	FREESTYLE	8X150
07:45-07:55	SPRINT	FREESTYLE	10X50
07:55-08:00	COOL DOWN	OWN CHOICE	200

The table describes a swim training with a technique focus that describes my swimming training routine.

TIME	STAGE	TYPE	Distance (m)
07:00-07:15	WARM UP	OWN CHOICE	3X50
07:15-07:30	ENDURANCE	FREESTYLE	4X100, 4X50, 4X25
07:30-07:45	ENDURANCE	FREESTYLE	5X200
07:45-07:55	SPRINT	FREESTYLE	5X50
07:55-08:00	COOL DOWN	OWN CHOICE	200

The table describes a swim training with an endurance focus that describes my swimming training routine.

THE BENEFITS OF CYCLING

I remember vividly my first bike ride with my brand-new road race bike. On a Thursday evening in March 2022, in Amsterdam. In the Netherlands, March is still a cold month, the weather is chilly and windy, but the days are becoming longer, so I thought it could be a perfect occasion to test my new bike. I decided to show up at the beginner ride event organized by ATAC triathlon club. Shy and anxious, I showed up for a ride that was supposed to be for beginners. I was clueless on the group riding rules and how to be a good rider myself. I clearly remember my white cycling shoes, ordered online and never tried before, my cheap cycling bib that I would have discovered soon enough was not comfortable at all. Suggestions for the future, even though I was lucky, and my shoes were super comfy, do not order online that try the cycling shoes beforehand. Moreover, I learned on the go how to clip in and out from the fixed pedals, of course not without falling at least a couple of times.

The ATAC people were really nice, despite it being annoying for them to explain all the rules of safe cycling to a beginner like me. Finally, we took off! The ride was stressful on many points, but most of all, regarding my glucose management. At that time, my CGM was not updating me in real time; I had to extract my phone, move it close to my arm, activate the NFC and see the value on the screen. This procedure to check my blood glucose was extremely difficult for a beginner biker like me. Apart from being difficult, it was also dangerous to do while group riding. I learned the hard way to understand the hypoglycemia feeling my body was giving me, and I learned the hard way to integrate before it is too late.

That day everything went wrong and unfortunately, the sensor stopped working because of the cold. I felt the pressure of the group becoming tired and impatient. I explained that I had diabetes, but it is a disease not well understood in its deep mechanisms.

At that time, I was not only a beginner on the bike but also a beginner in managing glucose levels during hours of training. My glucose dropped as a new aerobic activity such as cycling required a higher energetic consumption. Many lessons were learned from that day: Make sure to bring with me glucagon spray, carry extra gels in the pockets and cover the CGM sensor with extra layers as it is sensitive to the cold. I learned that it is better not to rely on technology and always bring the machine to perform the old school blood glucose test. Moreover, as today, before the start I would inform my biking friends regarding my chronic condition, and I would give them some dextrose tables to support me in case of a hypoglycemic event.

Cycling is a highly effective cardiovascular exercise that, like swimming, improves insulin sensitivity and aids in glucose regulation. The sustained physical activity involved in cycling helps muscles take up glucose, reducing blood sugar levels and promoting better overall glycemic control. After swimming, biking is my second favorite cardiovascular exercise, as it allows me to relax and distract myself from anxious thoughts. I could bike for hours without having hard repercussions on my joints. After my slipped disk and left knee meniscus injury I found biking a peaceful place to hide and meditate on life uncertainties and challenges.

During the winter months, I train with my indoor trainer at home or at the local gym. My gym offers different options such as using the watt-bikes, indoor bikes with a power meter or join spinning lessons. This is great because I do not have to suffer and endure the cold training outside, but I can have the same results while staying fit and having fun with others. In summer, during those few weeks of sun in the Netherlands, I go outside for bike rides.

Cycling at different intensities and durations directly influences my blood glucose. During these years of practice, I realized it is possible to control my blood sugar using different strategies.

On the fifth of March 2022, I was ready to challenge myself with a bike ride. Every weekend the length of the bike ride changed together with the weather conditions; very windy, less windy, rainy or cloudy and cold. All these variables influence the glucose values and glucose management. I went outside cycling from 10:30 am to 13:00 pm (Graph 6). I had breakfast around 8:30 am, and I injected one unit of insulin at 8:00 am. The timing of the insulin injection, two to three hours before the exercise, has the aim to prevent hypoglycemia events, as the peak effect of the insulin would have been over. two slices of brown bread (80 grams), cereals with high protein content (40 grams) and a banana (30 grams) and two mandarins (30 grams). I clearly remember the anxiety and tension during my first bike rides, because of my lack of experience with the bike and lack of experience with diabetes management. Every bike ride is different, therefore I decided to track my effort with a scale from 1 to 10. That day, the bike ride had an intensity of 7 out of 10, a moderately high perceived effort. The graph on page 155 shows how the glucose remains stable during the whole activity and the hour afterwards. I considered this ride a successful result for my diabetes! I arrived home feeling really proud of myself and eager to start tracking my results. I hope sharing these stories will be an example of strength and determination but most of all an example of diabetes management.

The twelfth of March 2022 was a windy and cloudy day in Amsterdam. I looked outside the window, and my inner conflict regarding how to dress up for the bike ride started. I am never sure about how many layers I should wear, and I usually end up overdressing, as my dear biking friends know. Anyway, after pumping my tires and packing the snacks I left the house to go cycling from 10:00 am to 13:00 pm. Every bike ride is different, therefore I decided to keep tracking my effort with a scale from 1 to 10. The bike ride had a perceived effort of 8 out of 10. The conclusion from the following stories is that depending on the type of effort, the heart rate and the nutrition strategy my glucose will behave differently.

I had a nice rich breakfast around 8:30 am together with my morning coffee. The breakfast was composed of two slices of brown bread (80 grams), cereals with high protein content (40 grams) and a banana (30 grams). I have made sure two hours and a half passed from the start of the activity from the insulin injection. In this way I make sure to reduce the chances of hypoglycemia events as the fast-acting insulin effect is almost over. This bike ride had a higher intensity compared to the one shown in graph 6, I could feel it in my legs getting heavy and my breathing becoming difficult. After 40 min of riding, I felt the need to integrate with an energy gel, called RioVit. The CGM showed 150 mg/dL (8.3 mmoL/L), perfect glucose, but my feelings were telling me otherwise. In the end, I always trust my feelings. I recognized this body sensation as a hypoglycemia event coming soon, therefore I had a gel, I promptly extracted it from my back pocket. I kept pushing on the ride, finishing with a glucose around 5.0 mmoL/L (90 mg/dL).

This would have been a difficult situation for me to handle if the ride had been longer, probably I would have needed to start integrating with an additional gel sooner. For this adventure another success! Diabetes 0, Eleonora 1!

On the twenty sixth of March 2022, I joined a 60 km ride starting from 9:30 am to 12:30 pm. This time the bike ride had a perceived effort of 8 out of 10. As planned, I enjoyed my lovely breakfast around 8:30 am, and I injected 1 unit of insulin around 8:00 am. I used the same nutrition strategy described, two slices of brown bread (80 grams), cereals with high protein content (40 grams) and a banana (30 grams), but this time the graph shows a glucose spike. What happened before the ride? Biking to the meeting point, I felt unwell and quite weak, therefore I made the quick decision to have some chocolate. That piece of chocolate gave me a sense of tranquility, despite noticing my glucose spiking up. I held myself not to react and in fact after 30 minutes, the glucose dropped. As I mentioned, the ride was quite demanding, and I started my integration with a SIS gel. At the time I was experimenting which gel would react best with my metabolism between RioVit, SIS and Gluc Up. Gluc Up gel was recommended to me by a diabetic marathon runner and guess what my conclusion was that Gluc Up gel containing only 15g Glucose is the best one for me. The Gluc up gel has the effect of increasing my glucose level in a controlled and stable way for the next hour.

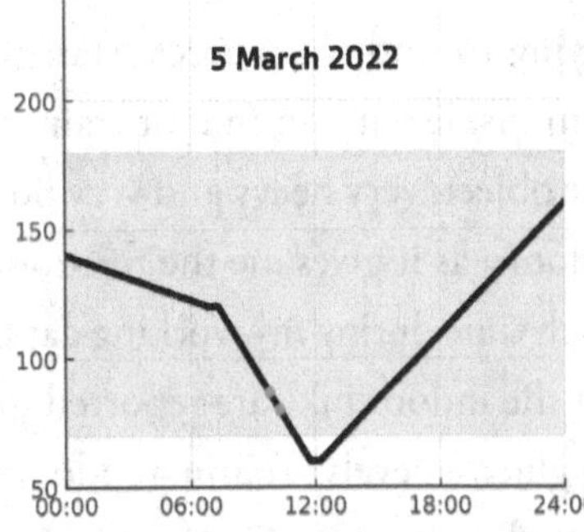

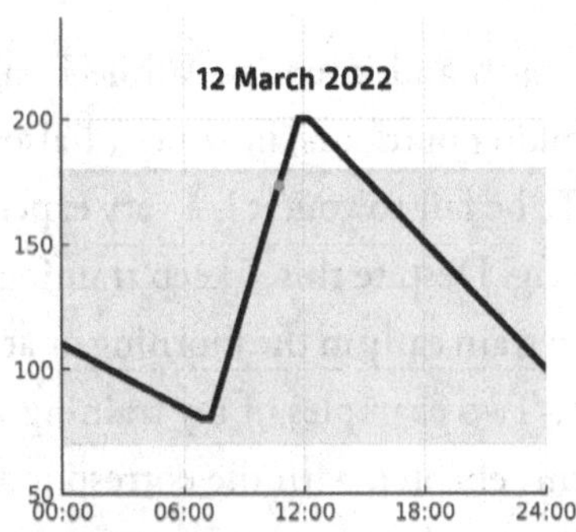

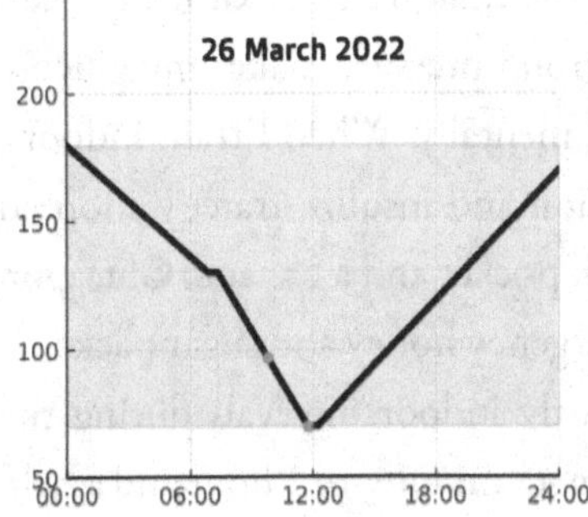

The graphs show the cycling sessions during March 2022. The cycling sessions varied in intensity, showing stable glucose levels after moderate-high rides on March 5th, a mid-ride glucose drop despite high-intensity efforts on March 12th, and a spike followed by recovery with glucose gel during a 60 km ride on March 26th.

My first bike rides were everything apart from easy to manage for my Diabetes, they were nightmares! I was experiencing every kind of sensation in my body and most of all they were all new feelings. I have never been on a bike for three or four or even six hours before. The body was in pain. I was asking "Why am I doing this?" The lower back hurt, my wrist hurt, and my glucose is absolutely going crazy, sharply up and sharply down. I had no idea of what I needed to eat to sustain hours of bike ride without diabetes, I could not imagine what to do with diabetes.

As I love challenges, I decided I wanted to perfect my glucose management during bike rides, so I started increasing progressively the length and intensity. While I am trying to find the perfect strategy biking outdoors, in winter, I also train inside with an indoor trainer. To be fair to you, it is a very expensive object, very heavy and very boring. Despite this, I keep training indoors, as it gives me the freedom to train early in the morning or at lunch time during my working days.

Two examples of my training with the indoor bike are reported in this chapter, with the corresponding glucose levels. Training indoors is easier in many aspects, in my personal experience. First, managing food and hydration is not an issue. The tranquility of knowing I can step off my bike anytime without group pressure makes my glucose more stable and plays a massive role mentally. When I train indoors, I make sure to have the same nutrition and insulin strategy adopted outdoors; a couple of gels in my back pocket and a banana. Glucagon spray always in my bike bag and emergency honey and sugar packs.

My training plan consists of mostly indoor intervals during the working week, short but intense from 45 minutes to 1 hour and a half. On the weekend, I train long distances from 70 km to 120 km.

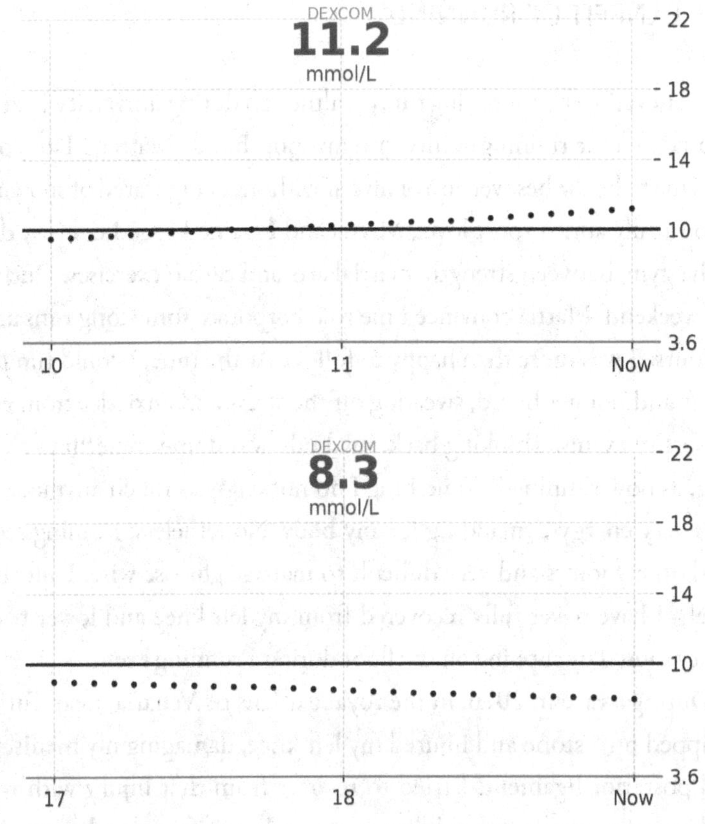

These graphs indicate the blood glucose concentration observed over 3-hours respective time periods respectively to the previous shown training. The first graph represents the half distance specific training while the other graph refers to the second training.

THE BENEFIT OF RUNNING

I have never been an amazing runner, although during university I participated in some running events with my sport buddy Mattia. Mattia pushed me to be the best version of myself without being scared of showing who I really am: A sport lover. Mattia and I trained together every day at the gym, between strength, martial arts and cardio exercises. During the weekend, Mattia convinced me to incorporate some long runs and of course I was more than happy to follow. At the time, I could run for hours and not get bored, sweating off the stress and anxieties from the university exams. Thinking back, my body was doing something amazing, as now running is something I do not enjoy as much anymore. It feels very energy demanding for my body. Nonetheless, running feels hard on my joints and very difficult to manage glucose wise. Unfortunately, I have never fully recovered from my left knee and lower back injury caused by slipping on the floor during a running event.

During a race in 2016, in the royal gardens of Venaria, near Turin, I slipped on a stone and injured my left knee, damaging my meniscus and posterior ligament. I tried to recover from that injury with rest and lots of strength and stability exercises, but unfortunately my knee did not fully recover. At the time, I decided not to go through surgery as with diabetes my recovery time and healing process would be potentially longer and more difficult. I had to stay still for several months, which also affected my lower back as I lost strength and developed a slipped disk in the lumbar area.

That year was physically devastating and emotionally challenging, but I learned to get back on my feet and start again. I never expected that I would be able to run again and join a triathlon team years later.

My message here is to keep trying, never give up and results will come eventually if you are fully dedicated. The motivation comes and goes but my strength is my discipline and commitment are always there. Time taught me to invest in myself as there is nothing more precious than my health.

Now, I am back to running twice a week. Before having a triathlon coach, I started learning as much as I could through books. One of my favorites is "Run faster the 5k to the Marathon" by Brad Hudson. One running session consists of hard and short intervals while the second session is a long and steady run. The mistake I see more often is that people run most of the time. The interval session is not hard enough while the long run session is often too fast instead of being an easy focused session. Since the beginning what I noticed about my glucose levels is that running tends to be a more energy-intensive exercise than swimming and biking. This means I need to adopt a different strategy for my diabetes management, and this requires time, mistakes and flexible adjustment.

According to literature, the energy consumption during running versus swimming and biking can vary depending on several factors, including the individual's weight, fitness level, intensity of the activity, and terrain.

Running training variations play a significant role in the glucose management, with factors such as the speed of running, the intensity of the workout, and the duration of the activity. These variables all influence energy consumption and, consequently, blood glucose levels.

I had multiple occasions to confront experiences with my triathlon friends, some of them may find running more demanding, while others may feel that biking requires more effort, that brought me to the conclusion that glucose consumption is very different from individual to individual.

For me, it is a different story, as my glucose management is more complex during running when I noticed I required more carbohydrates to sustain the activity compared to biking. I envy those light individuals with a typical running body, managing to run smoothly and effortlessly. Despite all my efforts, I have not achieved my top running performance, but there is still time to get there!

As I mentioned, I run twice a week: an interval run session on Wednesday and a long and steady run on Sunday. I love the running sessions because they turn into a moment to see my friends and push each other while catching up about life.

When I go for a run outside, I must carefully plan my nutrition and my insulin doses in the last three hours before the start. In my case, getting ready for running is not like in the Nike advertisement, just wear your shoes and run off, on the contrary, it is a long process before leaving the house. I make sure to have my running belt packed with insulin, sugar, gels and glucagon spray. I always run with my phone as it acts as my CGM. I learned from experience that the best thing to do would be to run as well with the finger glucose machine, just in case the CGM would fail.

Unfortunately, the heat and the cold can influence the readings and in my experience the difference between the blood test and the CGM could be more than 30%. This is particularly dangerous during physical activity, and many times I got scared about some false low glucose events, that forced me to integrate and stop. Therefore, my advice is always to bring the blood test machine.

Training with my triathlon team, Amsterdam Triathlon and Cycling (ATAC), not only gave me strength and positivity but also more knowledge into the running technique thanks to the presence of a running coach once a month.

Once I have improved my running technique, I started keeping track of how my glucose would increase or decrease depending on the training type and intensity. Improving my running skills, also stimulated me to increase my knowledge regarding the heart rate cardiac zones I experience while training.

The cardiac zone, often referred to as the heart rate zone, is a range of heart rates that correspond to different levels of exercise intensity. These zones are used to target specific fitness goals, such as improving cardio-vascular endurance, burning fat, or increasing aerobic capacity. Typically, heart rate zones are defined as a percentage of your maximum heart rate, which can be estimated by subtracting your age from 220.

After many and many tests and data collections, I have found some general glucose predictions while running. In my case, running at Tempo, usually defined as Zone 3, results in a slight decrease in blood glucose at first, followed by a glucose stability phase. As soon as I stop running, I experience a fast drop in blood sugar, that I usually tackle with a protein shake and if needed 15 grams of sugar. When I run in Zone 2, my glucose drops slowly but consistently during the run. Every 15 minutes I noticed a decrease of 1 mmoL/L (20 mg/dL). My integration in case of a long and steady run consists of assuming a Gluc Up gel containing 15 grams glucose every 30 minutes.

Once a week, I train at running intervals. The running intervals should be very intense, increasing the heart rate to Threshold usually defined as Zone 4. I have noticed that during high intensity mixed

ZONE	% OF MAXIMUM HEART RATE	DESCRIPTION
1	50-60%	Very light exercise, suitable for warm-ups and cool-downs
2	60-70%	Light exercise, ideal for building endurance and burning fat
3	70-80%	Moderate exercise enhances aerobic fitness and endurance, usually called "Tempo"
4	80-90%	Hard exercise improves cardiovascular capacity and anaerobic threshold, usually called "Threshold"
5	90-100%	Maximum effort, used for short bursts of high-intensity training to improve speed and power

The table shows the common heart rate zones from 1 to 5 with the % of the maximum heart rate and the description.

workout or anaerobic work the blood sugar spikes up suddenly by 30%. This happens as some stress hormones are released, increasing the blood sugar. In this case, I avoid integrating during the first 15 minutes and I wait until the end of the workout to correct with insulin or 15 grams of sugar if needed.

Regardless of what kind of interval or long run I am executing, my strategy is to keep checking my glucose and integrating every 30 minutes, if needed, with a banana or a Gluc up gel. I am very proud of my achievement of keeping my glucose stable when running long distances at a Zone 2 and Zone 3 pace, arriving at this point requires dedication and sacrifices but it is definitely possible for everyone who would like to achieve this result.

Here are some examples of running training I follow with explained my nutrition strategy and my glucose levels graphs. The running training on Sunday is usually two hours; from 10:00 am till 12:00 pm or from 14:00 pm till 16:00 pm. My nutrition strategy, two hours before the start, is: 30 grams of protein and 20 grams of long-lasting carbs such as a slice of brown bread. Most of the time, I try to play with the basal insulin and with the short acting insulin in order to have the minimum amount of active insulin when running, in order to avoid hypoglycemia events.

I will describe the following glucose graphs from left to right, explaining the key variables for glucose management during sport. The first graph represents a Zone 2 run with an integration of half a banana at 15:00 pm. In this graph I can conclude that I should have integrated earlier as my glucose drops quite fast in the next 30 minutes. Despite these remarks, I am happy with my glucose management for a Zone 2 run. Moving on to the second graph, this shows an interval running characterized by longer intervals at an effort 50% of the time at Zone 3 (tempo) and

50% at Zone 4 (Threshold) heart rate. This graph is less smooth, and it is not a straight flat line. On the contrary it is noticeable how the glucose increases for the first hours and then stabilizes it. This effect is typical of a zone 3 run (60% of the running time) and threshold run (40% of the running time). Another different scenario is in the last graph, that represents my glucose value during a threshold run in Zone 4. The glucose sharply increases due to the stress hormones released by the body.

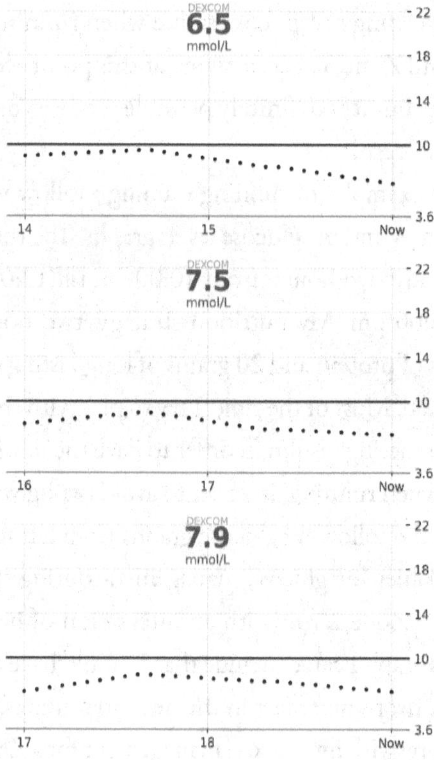

These graphs indicate the average blood glucose concentration observed over these respective time periods while running at different intensities, zone 2, zone 3, zone4.

RACE PREPARATION

Spring is in the air in the Netherlands! The sun is coming out, bringing me great joy inside. Longer and warmer days mean more time to train outside, finally having the chance to simulate a triathlon race. From my triathlon coach and my diabetologist I was advised to always try to simulate a race and never attempt a distance I have never done before as it could be dangerous for the glucose management.

A triathlon simulation is a structured and comprehensive practice session that mimics the conditions and challenges of an actual triathlon race. Triathlons typically consist of three segments: swimming, cycling, and running. The standard distances for each segment vary depending on the type of triathlon:

Sprint Triathlon
- Swim: 750 meters (0.47 miles)
- Bike: 20 kilometers (12.4 miles)
- Run: 5 kilometers (3.1 miles)

Olympic (Standard) Triathlon
- Swim: 1.5 kilometers (0.93 miles)
- Bike: 40 kilometers (24.8 miles)
- Run: 10 kilometers (6.2 miles)

Half Ironman (70.3)
- Swim: 1.9 kilometers (1.2 miles)
- Bike: 90 kilometers (56 miles)
- Run: 21.1 kilometers (13.1 miles, half marathon)

Ironman
- Swim: 3.8 kilometers (2.4 miles)
- Bike: 180 kilometers (112 miles)
- Run: 42.2 kilometers (26.2 miles, marathon)

Simulating a triathlon provides several benefits for athletes, including physical, mental, and logistical advantages. In my case, it is not only an advantage but a real need, as I need to be prepared for any possible glucose scenario.

Finishing my first Sprint was a huge satisfaction, a childhood dream that came true. Since a young age I always wanted to complete a triathlon with diabetes. In 1999, when I was diagnosed, people with diabetes were highly recommended not to practice sport, or at least to avoid high intensity as it could cause severe hypoglycemia.

Growing up, there was not too much knowledge about diabetes and sport in my diabetology clinic. Despite this I embarked on swimming competitions. During my teens, I left Italy with many uncertainties and doubts but with the hope to find more knowledge about diabetes and sport elsewhere. In the Netherlands, I decided to challenge myself with triathlons, and the first thing I did was to ask for support from the specialists in the local hospital.

The Dutch diabetologist was very surprised, looking at me like an alien. "Triathlon?! Wow, let me know how it goes and what you do to manage it." I was surprised and at the same time disappointed as I was looking for suggestions and advice myself, but that was not the case!

This episode pushed me even more to write down my experience, failures and progress, to share and inspire others that like me, would have loved guidance for their endurance sport challenge.

Preparing any kind of triathlon distance is not easy. Sprint triathlon is an easy distance, I always hear. Perhaps it is, if you do not have diabetes, but I can assure you that is not easy at all for me. Triathlons demand a high level of endurance but also a high level of understanding of your body. After completing five to ten sprint distances, I started simulating Olympic and Half Ironman distances, as I was ready to challenge my body to the next level.

A Half Ironman is not a joke for people without diabetes, so you can imagine how difficult and challenging it can be if you have a chronic condition directly impacting your nutrition, sport performance and mental state.

To arrive as prepared as possible for my main event, the Half Ironman event, I practiced double training such as bike-riding but also carefully planned and studied what to do in the transition moments. Optimizing transitioning is key for a diabetes T1 athlete has helped me optimize my routines, such as checking glucose, packing the glucagon spray and insulin on the bike, and ensuring all my nutrition is ready. Through simulations, I could fine-tune my nutrition plans, ensuring they have the right balance of carbohydrates, proteins, and fats to maintain stable blood glucose levels.

RACE SIMULATION

For athletes with diabetes, the glucose benefits of simulating a race or long training session are significant. By closely monitoring glucose levels during different segments of the triathlon simulation, I can gain experience and make the right adjustments to insulin doses, nutrition, and hydration plans. This proactive approach helps maintain stable blood glucose levels, preventing both hyperglycemia and hypoglycemia during the actual race (as much as possible). Moreover, this approach helped me create different strategy plans depending on the different glucose scenarios.

On the 20th of March 2022 and on the 11th of June 2022, as respectively represented in the pictures, I combined three sports together for the first time. This had the purpose to test if my body would be capable of handling a full triathlon fitness wise and try to understand how my glucose would react to such a long training window. The anxiety of the unknown was invading me. I was nervous, with cramps in my stomach, noticing a higher resting heart rate. The menu of the day was to do an inverse triathlon, running, biking, swimming. The planned exercise window was from 9:00 am till 14:00 pm. I woke up with hypoglycemia that concerned me, making me react with eating a fruit salad (35 grams of carbohydrates). Before the start of the run, as I was still in hypoglycemia, I ate four mandarins (48 grams carbohydrates). The glucose fluctuates from 8.9 mmoL/L (160 mg/dL) up to 12.5 mmoL/L (220 mg/d) then slowly back to 7.2 mmoL/L (130 mg/dL) after running exercise. During the exercise I integrated with 30 grams of long-lasting carbohydrates (100 grams of integral bread) resulting in a glucose spike at 12:00 pm. Before and after swimming, I made sure to integrate with proteins, eating three eggs.

To be the first time attempting a full triathlon, I was happy with my results! Most of all, I knew I had the right positive mindset, absorbing every moment as a positive learning experience. The aim of this first try out was not to focus on distance and performance but on glucose management. What I would do differently next time is to avoid such a fast sugar release food for breakfast and reduce by 20% the carbohydrate integration at 11:30 am. Moreover, I will avoid eating eggs before swimming as I found them hard to digest in such a short time.

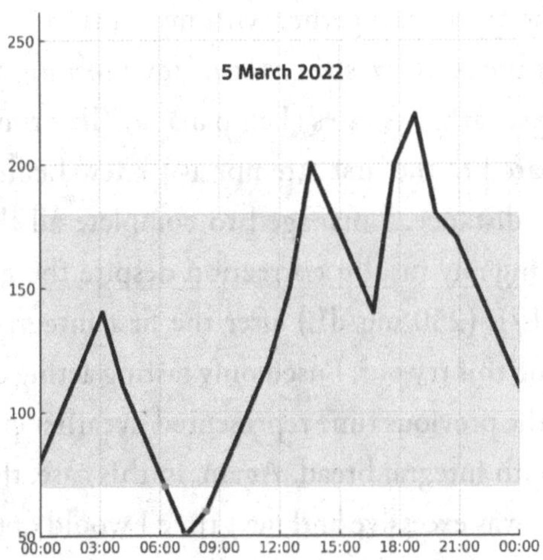

This graph shows the glucose levels at different times of the day during my test triathlon.

TIME	VALUE 1	NUTRITION	SPORT	VALUE 2	INSULIN
9:45	50 MG/DL	4 MANDARINS	RUN 60MIN	160 MG/DL	NO INSULIN
11:00	120 MG/DL	100GR BREAD	BIKE 20MIN	120 MG/DL	
13:00	150 MG/DL	3 EGGS	SWIM 30MIN	220 MG/DL	-
14:00	-	3 EGGS	-	130 MG/DL	-

The table shows the three sports I practiced on 20th of March. The table tracks the eating and insulin doses administered.

On the 11th of June 2022, I attempted to combine three different sports in a day for the second time. This time I changed the sequence to bike, run and swim. The day before I had planned the start of the activity at 11:00 am. I scheduled my breakfast two hours before the start of the exercise, together with my morning insulin dose. A protein-based breakfast was the star of my morning together with 30 grams of fast carbohydrates (half banana). This time, I was more relaxed compared to the first attempt as I knew I could have brought home the distance. I managed to complete all three activities without needing any insulin correction despite the glucose spiked to 13.9 mmoL/L (250 mg/dL) after the first integration of half a banana. During this try out, I used only fasting acting carbohydrates compared to the previous time represented in earlier example, where I integrated with integral bread. Again, in this case, the integration of half banana was excessive and next time I would opt for a smaller amount of it.

I arrived home devastated; I could barely walk up the steep Dutch stairs leading to my apartment door. Given hyperglycemia I injected three units of insulin, resulting in a fast glucose drop in less than one hour. Reflecting on my glucose graph, I noticed that after a long day of activity my glucose was more prone to fast decrease. Physical activity enhances insulin sensitivity, meaning the body's cells are more responsive to insulin. This increased sensitivity can persist for hours to even days after exercise, causing glucose to be taken up by the cells more efficiently, leading to lower blood glucose levels.

Managing glucose levels with type 1 diabetes requires careful monitoring and adjustment of insulin doses, particularly after periods of physical activity. It is crucial to recognize these factors and adjust dietary intake, insulin administration, and activity levels accordingly to maintain optimal glucose control.

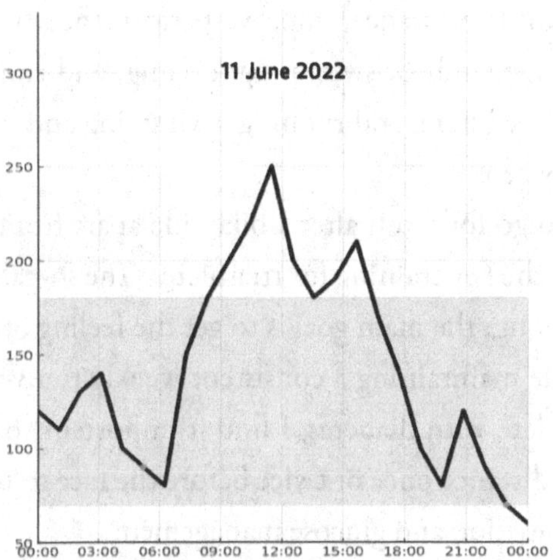

This graph shows the glucose levels at different times of the day during my "try out" triathlon on June 11, 2022. I successfully combined three sports activities starting at 11:00 am

TIME	1ST GLUCOSE VALUE	NUTRITION	SPORT	2ND GLUCOSE LEVEL	INSULIN
11:00 AM	150 MG/DL	BANANA	BIKE 50KM	250MG/DL	NO INSULIN
13:00 PM	160 MG/DL	SIS GEL	RUN 5KM	220MG/DL	-
14:00 PM		APPLE	SWIM 2KM	130MG/DL	-

The table shows the three sports I practiced on 11th of June. The table shows the glucose level before and after, the nutrition and insulin doses administered.

DOUBLE TRAINING

Triathletes practice double training, meaning not only exercising twice a day, to build endurance, improve performance, and adapt their bodies to the demands of swimming, cycling, and running. Double training could be biking and running, swimming and biking without a break in between.

Deciding to go for a run after a bike ride apart from being exhausting is one of the key training for triathletes. The so-called brick runs are never too long; the main goal is to get the feeling of running with tired legs while maintaining a consistent weekly run volume. However, as a triathlete with diabetes, I find it important to complete the full brick run distance once or twice before the race to test something specific like nutrition and glucose management.

The graph on the next page represents a double training (Bike-Run) session on the 28th of April 2024. I was biking from 9:00 am till 11:00 pm and running from 11:30 pm till 13:30 pm. To stretch and relax I concluded the brick session with 30 minutes of yoga. Let's start with my nutrition strategy during breakfast. It included 30 grams of slow carbohydrates and 20 grams of protein. The protein helps keep the glucose stable, flattening the glucose spike that carbohydrates would create.

I started with a glucose level of 3.9 mmoL/L (70 mg/dL), and by the end of the bike ride, my glucose was back at 4.4 mmoL/L (80 mg/dL). I did not feel the need of any integration until the end of the bike ride when I had a protein bar. The run was at an easy pace, Zone 2. During the run I integrated Gluc Up gel every 30 minutes.

I started incorporating double training sessions more frequently, after one year of practicing triathlon training. At the beginning I was focused on surviving one hard training a day, while after a year, I became more confident with my diabetes management in each of the singular sports. The combination of cycling and running, trains the body to efficiently switch between different energy systems, optimizing the use of glucose and reducing the likelihood of sharp blood sugar spikes or drops.

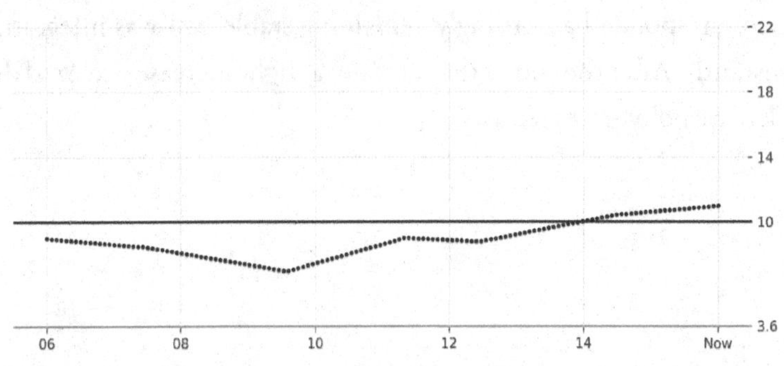

This graph shows the blood glucose level over a period of 6 hours during the double training bike-run session.

Another type of double training, I practice, is swimming and biking, represented in the following picture. Swim-bike training helps me understand how my glucose fluctuates from swimming to biking as this is the first part of a triathlon. Understanding how my body responds to the demands of consecutive activities, allows me to anticipate and adjust insulin doses and carbohydrate intake to prevent hypoglycemia or hyperglycemia during and after exercise.

Practicing bike-run or swim-bike helped me develop strategies for maintaining glucose control throughout the different stages of a triathlon. The picture shows my glucose level on a Sunday morning, where I went swimming indoors at 7:00 am at a local swimming pool, just five minutes away from my house. After swimming 2000 meters in about 40 minutes, I used my indoor bike trainer to train for another 45 minutes to one hour. The total workout ended around 9:30 am.

My nutrition strategy involved the use of a Gluc Up gel (15 grams of glucose) every 30-40 minutes as the effort was easy but steady. The glucose responded accordingly, remaining stable, as I was integrating constantly. After the end of the activities a slight increase occurred due to late carbohydrates release.

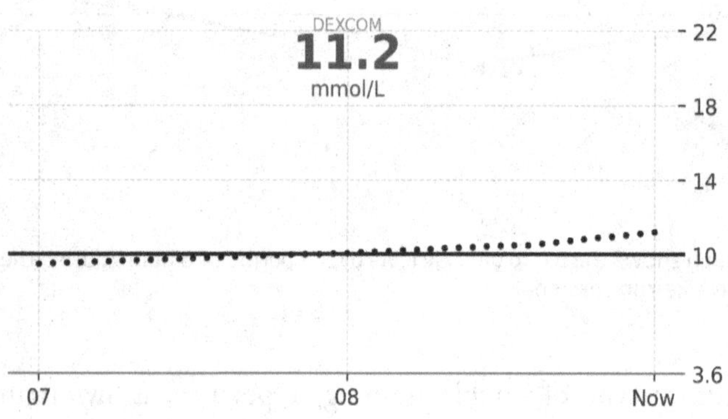

This graph shows the blood glucose level fluctuation over a period of 3 hours during my swim-bike training.

TRACKING PERFORMANCE

Seems prehistoric, but I remember times when a little paper book was handed out at the diabetology clinic to facilitate the patients in tracking their glucose data. The old school pen and paper, completely replaced now by the CGM apps. Tracking the progress in diabetes management is crucial and very beneficial but can be stressful both using apps or pen and paper! I noticed that for me the constant vigilance and detailed record-keeping required can be overwhelming and anxiety-inducing. The need to balance insulin, food, and physical activity demands continual attention and can be mentally exhausting.

What helped me in this journey was the drive to share my experience and my diabetes management details in order to help others. Accurate monitoring of my blood glucose levels, my insulin doses, and carbohydrate intake helped me to identify patterns and make necessary and more precise adjustments to maintain stable glucose levels.

Keeping track of my progress in both performance and glucose management has been crucial for achieving glucose stability while also improving my athletic performance. First and foremost, having a standardized and optimized nutrition strategy allowed me to understand how different efforts affect my glucose levels. I use a nutrition and sports app called Lifesum, where I log my nutrition and physical activity every day. Using the app made me become more aware of what I eat, and I started reflecting on how my glucose level was influenced by that before and after training. During the last years, I have not always managed to focus on performance without getting worried, stressed, paranoid towards my glucose levels and a key helper was my nutritionist who encouraged me to keep training no matter what. He encouraged me to liberate myself from the constant checking of the glucose levels and focus on training, partially setting aside the stress of glucose variability.

Thanks to the nutritionist's suggestion I started keeping track of my progress. To do so, I use two apps such as Strava and Garmin Connect. These apps monitor my fitness and personal best times and efforts in swimming, running, and cycling for different distances. Mentally, tracking my progress provides a sense of accomplishment and motivation. Seeing positive changes in my performance and/or glucose levels stability while training boosts my confidence and encourages me to continue making healthy choices. On the other hand, if challenges arise, keeping track of my glucose and sport helps me pinpoint areas for improvement and empowers me to make informed decisions about my health.

For my learning process regarding how sport influences glucose behavior, it was important to slow myself down into pushing to achieve better performance results and deeply understand the thinking process behind reaching the desired glucose values.

Since I started practicing sports, the evolution of technology, already helped me to optimize my blood sugar control. Regular monitoring of blood glucose levels with a CGM, changed my life as before I was using a finger blood test. Using CGM I started becoming aware of glucose spikes after eating certain foods and possible drops during endurance physical activity. The second step into improving my sport and diabetes management was adjusting insulin doses based on these insights. Reducing the amount of insulin 3 hours before physical activity helped me maintain stable blood glucose levels, preventing both hyperglycemia and hypoglycemia. The third step involved understanding how my body responds to specific foods and how it responds to those foods during exercise routines. Finding the best strategy takes time, requires flexibility, and involves a process of small attempts, failures, and eventual success.

During my journey, I understood that having a solid foundation in nutrition strategy and sports knowledge is essential for achieving sports results. I started tracking my performance results once I had a fixed strategy for nutrition, allowing me to focus solely on performance.

My suggestion is to use a nutrition app to log the food and sports such as My Fitness Pal, Dally or Life Sum. If you are nostalgic about the old times, pen and paper will do the job perfectly.

17. MY PERFORMANCE TEST

One year into my triathlon journey, I felt the urge to deep dive into my performance data. First of all, I consulted my diabetologist looking for guidance and support into the performance and diabetes world. Unfortunately, the doctor did not have any experience with diabetes and triathlon, asking me to keep him updated on my glucose strategies and performance achievement. Deciding to seek advice elsewhere, I followed the suggestion of my nutritionist and my triathlon coach, keeping track of my performance. The tool to do so is with a performance test for swimming, biking, and running. The test involved a structured approach to evaluate current fitness level and identify areas for improvement. Here's a step-by-step guide I used:

- **Set Clear Goals:** Define what I want to achieve with the performance test, such as assessing endurance, speed, or technique.
- **Establish Baselines:**
  - **Swimming:** Time myself over a set distance (e.g., 400 meters) in a controlled environment. Noting down stroke count and technique.
  - **Biking:** Perform a time trial over a standard distance (e.g., 20 kilometers) on a consistent course. Record your time, average speed, and heart rate.
  - **Running:** Conduct a timed run over a known distance (e.g., 5 kilometers). Tracked my time, pace, and heart rate.

- **Warm-Up Properly:** I begin each test with a proper warm-up to prevent injury and ensure my best performance. I include light aerobic activity and dynamic stretches.
- **Execute the Test:** I maintain a consistent effort throughout each test.
- **Record Data:** I write down all relevant data immediately after each test, including times, heart rates, perceived effort, and any other observations.
- **Analyze Results:** I compare the performance against previous tests or establish benchmarks. This helps me to identify strengths and areas needing improvement.
- **Repeat Regularly:** I conduct these performance tests periodically (e.g., every 4-6 weeks) to monitor progress and make necessary adjustments to my training regimen.

The picture summarizes my performance metrics for swims, bike, and runs, repeated every 4-6 weeks in a five-month timeline.

My performance test could be defined as a field test, as I selected a benchmark, it is easy to execute and consequently easily repeatable. In order to execute correctly a field testing, it is necessary to be fully rested and push to the max effort.

This exercise not only helped me in becoming aware of my body capabilities but encouraged me to reflect on my performance. The result highlights improvements in swimming and running time. That was great to notice. Even though I considered myself a relatively good swimmer, I was proud to be able to push my limits. A pleasant surprise was to see that my biking average speed increased over time, encouraging me to keep up the good work. The following list is what I made sure to do:

- Pick a swimming distance (e.g., 200 m), running distance (e.g., 5 km), and biking segment (e.g., 20 km).
- Record time every month.
- Include glucose details before and after exercise.
- Nutrition information before and after.

DATE	SWIM DIST.	SWIM TIME	BIKE DIST.	BIKE AVG SPEED	RUN DIST.	RUN TIME
15 MAY 22	800 METERS	16 MIN.	20KM	25KM/H	5KM	30 MIN.
21 JUN 22	800 METERS	14 MIN.	20KM	35KM/H	5KM	26 MIN.
20 AUG 22	800 METERS	13 MIN.	20KM	35KM/H	5KM	25 MIN.
17 SEP 22	800 METERS	12 MIN.	20KM	30KM/H	5KM	25 MIN.

The table shows my performance metric of swim, bike, run over time.

DATA ANALYSIS

This table reflects a consistent improvement in the performance metrics for swimming, biking, and running over the specified dates. The swim times show a marked improvement from 16 minutes in May to 12 minutes in September, indicating enhanced efficiency and endurance in swimming. The bike ride demonstrates an increase in average speed from 25 km/h to 35 km/h between May and August, although there was a slight decrease to 30 km/h in September, which could be due to varying conditions or fatigue. The run times improved significantly from 30 minutes in May to 25 minutes in both August and September, reflecting better speed and stamina. These results suggest a positive trend in overall fitness and performance, showcasing progress and adaptation to training regimens. Each test provides valuable insights into physical conditioning, endurance, and speed, contributing to a comprehensive understanding of athletic performance over time.

The previous picture, does not keep track of the glucose levels and nutritional insight during the performance test, although I use an app for it called LifeSum. I just discovered that a CGM app such as Dexcom G7 gives the possibility to log insulin bolus, food and exercise.

If you would like to give a try in tracking your performance, use the tables in the next page.

Looking ahead, the integration of data analysis and AI tools offers a promising future for revolutionizing diabetes management. Imagine a groundbreaking tool that becomes indispensable for people with diabetes—a comprehensive system that consolidates data from various sources into a unified platform. This tool would integrate glucose values, insulin doses, heart rate (both minimum and maximum), heart rate variability, resting heart rate, oxygenation levels, blood pressure, breathing patterns, menstrual cycle phases, and hormone levels. Such a 360-degree approach could uncover correlations and patterns previously hidden, offering deeper insights into the multifaceted interactions affecting glucose management. By shifting the perspective from isolated data points to a holistic view, this tool could empower individuals to make informed decisions, personalize treatments, and improve outcomes. The potential to identify how these factors interplay might not only enhance diabetes care but also redefine how the

DATE	SWIM (KM)	TIME (MIN)	GLUCOSE VALUE (BEFORE)	NUTRITION	GLUCOSE VALUE (AFTER)

DATE	BIKE (KM)	TIME (MIN)	GLUCOSE VALUE (BEFORE)	NUTRITION	GLUCOSE VALUE (AFTER)

DATE	RUN (KM)	TIME (MIN)	GLUCOSE VALUE (BEFORE)	NUTRITION	GLUCOSE VALUE (AFTER)

This table can be used to track training combined with pre-run, pre-swim, pre-bike nutrition, and glucose levels.

condition is understood. With this vision, we could move beyond conventional diabetes management, paving the way for innovative solutions that bridge technology and health.Looking ahead, the integration of data analysis and AI tools offers a promising future for revolutionizing diabetes management. Imagine a groundbreaking tool that becomes indispensable for people with diabetes—a comprehensive system that consolidates data from various sources into a unified platform. This tool would integrate glucose values, insulin doses, heart rate (both minimum and maximum), heart rate variability, resting heart rate, oxygenation levels, blood pressure, breathing patterns, menstrual cycle phases, and hormone levels. Such a 360-degree approach could uncover correlations and patterns previously hidden, offering deeper insights into the multifaceted interactions affecting glucose management. By shifting the perspective from isolated data points to a holistic view, this tool could empower individuals to make informed decisions, personalize treatments, and improve outcomes. The potential to identify how these factors interplay might not only enhance diabetes care but also redefine how the condition is understood. With this vision, we could move beyond conventional diabetes management, paving the way for innovative solutions that bridge technology and health.

18. COMPETITIONS HISTORY

TRIAMSTERDAM

Tri Amsterdam is a very popular triathlon in Amsterdam. It usually hosts around two thousand people. The morning of the 19th of June 2022, my stomach was cramping from anxiety. Finally, here we are, the moment I have waited for so long, the dream coming true, the start.

At the time, I knew very little regarding the influence of stress or menstrual hormones on my glucose, nor I was confident on my nutrition strategy on my first triathlon. Everything was a big new challenge!

The night before, I did not sleep properly, nightmares of me not managing to cross the finishing line were all over my head. I woke up thirsty and nervous and I corrected the high glucose during the night with insulin. I fell back asleep, and I woke up ready to rock my first triathlon!

The dinner before the race was rich in carbohydrates as from the textbook. As it is common knowledge between athletes and I learned myself, I was supposed to do the famous "carb load" before a race. I was skeptical in following this guideline as I usually follow a low carb diet. In order to deal with a dinner rich in carbohydrate I resulted in injecting a higher dose of insulin, according to my insulin to carb ratio. Despite this, hyperglycemia events occurred during the night.

Unfortunately, I woke up many times, resulting in not being well rested in the morning. Every mistake, every challenge comes with a lesson learned. This time I learned to never try a nutrition or insulin strategy never tested and perfected, the evening before the race. It seems like obvious advice, but I saw for myself how many times I get tempted to copy what others do or rely on other advice and experience. From this experience I learned to seek professional advice before every decision I take.

Discussing with experts what I should have done as a nutrition strategy instead of the carbohydrate load, I learned that perhaps, a better strategy would be the one to progressively increase the amount of carbohydrates during the three days before the race.

Race day! I had carefully prepared all my equipment the night before; swimming goggles, caps, biking gear, running gear and I was surprised at how much equipment needed to be carried! Biking to the starting point, around 10 kilometers from my house, seems already challenging with all that weight on my back. My hands were shaking, my stomach was contracting. "You are ready for this" I was repeating to myself.

Despite trying to convince myself that I was ready for this challenge I knew that probably I was not, as it was the first time trying to manage my glucose during a triathlon. In order to facilitate my diabetes management, I had a nutrition strategy in place. My breakfast had some long-lasting carbohydrates such as rice biscuit and 20 grams of protein. Afterwards, my planned integration was to have a SIS gel every 30 minutes.

Here I am, at the start of the race. Perfect, the glucose before the start was exactly what I wanted. I left all my belongings to the bike transition, including the glucose monitor and my phone. This was the last time I could check my glucose before and during the swim, and this feeling gave me anxiety.

If you're wondering why I felt anxious and not liberated to be without my continuous glucose monitor (CGM) is because it became the safety net that keeps me steady. It's my version of Linus' blanket, offering me a sense of security that's hard to describe. With real-time updates on my glucose levels, I can catch trends before they become dangerous, whether I'm exercising, eating, or simply going about my day. Without it, I feel lost, relying on finger stick tests that only give me a momentary snapshot, leaving me anxious about what's happening in between.

For the final hour before the start, I had to rely on my feelings regarding the glucose fluctuation, but I was determined to complete this challenge, nothing could have stopped me.

A gunshot marked the rolling start for the swim. Jumping into the Amstel canal water was a pleasant experience only after the first 200 meters where I was punched and kicked by competitors. I discovered afterwards that this is normal in triathlons, and I should be more mindful of it.

I got out of the water, where I did not forget to smile at the photographer rushing to check my glucose. Unexpectedly it was very high, above 300 mg/dL (16 mmoL/L). Wow I was very surprised, wondering how possible such an increase was possible. I had a couple of split seconds to decide what to do, resulting into avoiding correcting the hyperglycemia. Couple of minutes later, I was out of the transition area, already on my bike. The legs felt heavy during the bike ride, the shoulder and the lower back were now painful as well. For a moment I wondered why I decided to do something like this, as I was not having fun at all. In a split second, this dark thought was gone, and I was bac at the transition area. The glucose did not decrease while riding, so I decided to inject 1 unit of insulin.

Another big surprise was to see that the glucose did not go down during the run, despite the active insulin in my body! Wow, the power of adrenaline and cortisol is very strong.

I crossed the finishing line with lots of joy but with a tired feeling as my glucose was at 300 mg/dL (16 mmoL/L) for the entire race. My legs were full of lactic acid, fatiguing in breathing. After celebrating, I managed to return to the transition area where I injected 3 units. It took the insulin 2 hours to make the glucose return to normal level.

Finally, the celebration moment with my Amsterdam and Cycling Triathlon friends. A rewarding and filling dinner made the glucose spike up again, because I was conservative on the unit of insulin administered to prevent hypoglycemia after exercise. This decision came because after sport the insulin sensitivity increases for several hours.

I could not fall asleep that evening, I was going through the race over and over again. As soon as I closed my eyes, I saw bikes sprinting next to me. I took some time to reflect on what I had done. I felt proud and brave. I felt accomplished, but not fully. Something was missing. I wanted to share my story for the first time. I felt the urge to tell how hard it is to face a triathlon with diabetes and how beautiful it is to finish one. I felt the need to share the details of my race from a diabetes point of view because someone out there, like me, would like to attempt it one day. The race atmosphere is such a unique experience, that diabetes cannot be a roadblock!

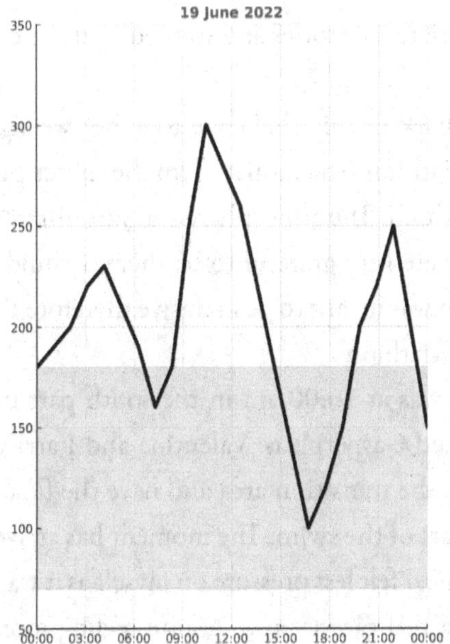

The graph shows the glucose levels during the Amsterdam Triathlon on the 19th of June 2022.

SLOW TRIATHLON

Now to the next Triathlon! In August 2022, I participated in an Olympic distance triathlon with my friend Valentina. I met Vale attending an open water swimming course. The teacher, Michiel, an amazing swimmer, taught us how to navigate in open water and how to overcome the challenges possibly arising in an open water race. Vale immediately became my friend because her smile and happiness were just contagious. After 6 weeks of open water courses together, she got interested in my triathlon stories and wanted to try to complete a triathlon herself.

Excited to embark in this challenge together we signed ourselves up for a charity triathlon. The money from the subscription was donated for cancer research. The atmosphere was just different, calmer. All the participants were very grateful to be there, I could see it in their eyes. The triathlon was meant to be inclusive therefore the name of the event was "Slow Triathlon".

The start time was at 10:00 am in the south part of Amsterdam, around a lake called Gasperplaas. Valentina and I arrived early to arrange the bikes in the transition area and have the final food integration before the start of the swim. The moment has arrived, off I go for the swim. This time, I felt less pressure on myself as it was a fundraising event instead of a real race event. Despite feeling more at ease, and despite a smooth and fast swim, my glucose spiked up again.

After 1500-meter swimming, I jumped out of the water full of energy with a big smile on my face. Arriving at the transition, the glucose values were a bit higher than expected but I decided not to inject any insulin to correct the hyperglycemia. I felt strong on the bike, leading the way. 40 km with Valentina passed so fast, even though the bike ride lasted 1 hour and 40 min. During the bike ride I kept going, integrating with a sip of SIS gel, every 30 minutes.

I changed my shoes, I packed my back pockets with gels, and I was ready to face the most challenging part of an Olympic triathlon, the run. The 10 kilometers run was a mix of walk and run, together with Valentina. We wanted to stick together till the end. My glucose kept staying high during the full race and as a side effect my legs started being more fatigued and my breathing was heavy. Despite this challenge I crossed the finish line. There was not a medal in the end but a stunning flower to symbolize the beauty of the life we are living!

After the race, I refueled with protein and carbohydrates. The insulin I injected after the race made my glucose drop faster than usual as the insulin effect is amplified after physical activity due to increased insulin sensitivity, enhanced muscle glucose uptake, and the body's need to replenish glycogen stores.

I was scared by this huge drop that made me feel tired and dizzy suddenly. My lesson learned for this race is to be careful with the insulin I inject after the race and be more conscious about delayed drops in glucose levels. Eleonora 1-Diabetes 0!

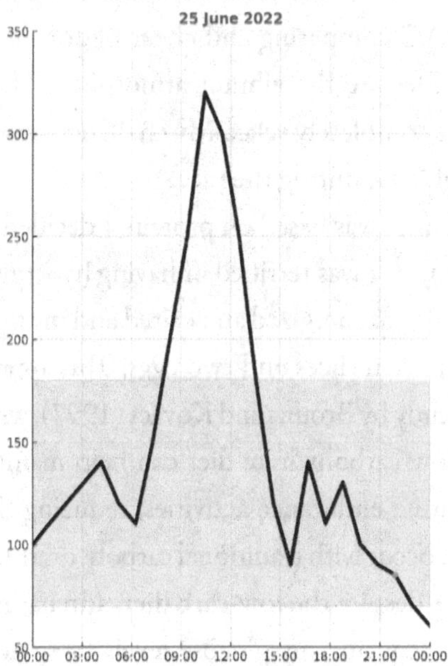

The graph shows my glucose management on the 19th of August 2022 Olympic triathlon with Valentina.

TRIATHLON OUDEKERK

One of my best performance triathlons was Oudekerk. Oudekerk is a small town near Amsterdam. During this triathlon I wanted to push my mind and my body and so I did. I had an optimized nutrition strategy, and I was confident I could do the sprint distance easily. I was very happy about my swim results of 12:58 minutes. On the bike I felt strong. As usual the wind is never lacking in the Netherlands, forcing me to bike against the wind for 35 minutes. Despite the tiredness after the bike ride, I ran my third best 5km!

The pre-race atmosphere in Oudekerk was fantastic, making me forget about the stress of the competition. During the race, I saw someone from ATAC competing and cheering for me, which gave me positive energy. Despite the vibrant atmosphere, the cheer and laughter I could not completely relax. My challenge was as always to manage my blood glucose during the race.

My evening dinner was based on protein. I decided to avoid the carbohydrates loading as I was terrified of having hyperglycemia all through the night. I woke up energized and exited and my breakfast consisted of 30 grams of chicken slices and two eggs. This approach aligns with findings from a study by Brouns and Kovacs (1997), which suggests that a high-protein, low-carbohydrate diet can help maintain stable blood glucose levels during endurance activities, reducing the risk of hyperglycemia that can occur with traditional carbohydrate loading strategies.

Unfortunately, despite the low-carb diet, adrenaline played a significant role, again, causing my glucose levels to spike. Despite this, I started with reasonable glucose levels, but as soon as I got into the water, I noticed a huge and fast increase.

Every race is a learning moment. From this one, I learned to address rising glucose levels sooner, as I now understand the impact of adrenaline.

TRIATHLON BOOSBAN

Amsterdam Triathlon and Cycling club organizes a member only group race after the summer holiday. After spending my vacation time in Italy, I returned to the Netherlands where the weather was miserable. I was missing my family, the food and the sun. This was my mood on the 17th of September 2022. I felt sad and tired, and to be honest I didn't even want to show up. I decided to get out of bed and make the most of it. My race plan was simple: bring home the swim, have fun biking, and survive the run.

I followed all the advice discussed during previous calls with my nutritionist such as avoid carbohydrate loading the night before, correcting hyperglycemia, injecting insulin after the swim and try not to get stressed. Most of all, try to enjoy the day!

First of all, I woke up three hours before the race and managed to have a nice relaxing breakfast. My plan was working as I injected 1 unit of insulin beforehand—something I hadn't done previously. Usually, I wait till the swim is completed to inject 1 or 2 units. My bike, my bag and my mindset were ready to race now. Arriving at the starting location, I felt butterflies in my stomach and a huge feeling of gratitude. My body is about to do something amazing again, despite diabetes.

Here we go, it's time to go to the starting area. I left my phone, which allows me to see my CGM data, in the transition area. I was confident my glucose would stay stable but this time I was less sure as I injected 1 unit for breakfast. To be safe, I carry with me 1 gel in the back pocket of the Tri suit, in case of hypoglycemia during the swim.

I swam as fast as I could, with an expected threshold heart rate. Coming out of the swim I felt dizzy, sitting down I checked my glucose, and I injected 1 unit of insulin to prevent my glucose from spiking too high during the bike ride. The bike ride was tough as the course contained 4 sharp turns and windy roads. Additionally, before the run, I injected 2 more units. The performance results were good despite my glucose values being not so astonishing; my glucose did not drop below 250 mg/dL (13.9 mmoL/L) for the entire two hours and kept rising for another hour after the race finished.

MY TRIATHLON PERFORMANCE

The swim was one of my best times! 10 minutes for 750 meters. I came out of the water second!

The run was also a success! 5 kilometers in 25 minutes.

After the race, I injected 4 units to make the glucose drop. I have observed that, given the presence of adrenaline and cortisol hormone, the insulin effect was reduced, and it took longer than usual to decrease the glucose levels.

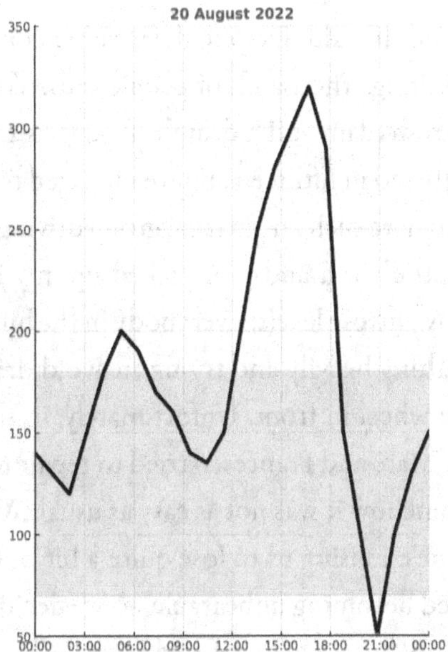

The glucose graph shows the glucose levels the evening before the race (Sat) and the race day (Sun).

BIKE RACE

The Netherlands has a lot of bike races throughout the country, one of the most famous is the DAM to DAM, meaning "City to City." This race is held in September in Amsterdam. The month of September can be really frustrating as the rain is unpredictable and where there is incessant rain. That morning the weather forecast was terrible, but I was determined to ride for this race, as also my father came all the way from Italy for it. I showed up at the race start with a rain jacket, arm warmers, and leg warmers, and even with a cap below the helmet to be ready to endure the cold and the rain. Despite the weather conditions, the start of the race was exciting. Thousands of people gathered in Dam Square, in the heart of Amsterdam and a drum roll gave us the start sign. My triathlon club gathered in fifthteen and we managed to ride for 150km. I was very lucky to have such an amazing group driving me forward.

Soon enough, the wind and rain picked up, my body stress kept rising as well as my glucose levels. Everybody in the bike pack had their head down, breathing heavily and trying to avoid drinking the water sprayed from the wheel in front. Unfortunately, in the cold and rain we had a flat tire. Marc and Francesco tried to repair Marc's flat as fast as possible but somehow it was not as easy as usual. We stopped in the cold for 20 minutes, causing us to lose quite a bit of body heat. Cold and fatigue started becoming unbearable, so we decided to try to stop in a bar to warm up, but we were refused entry. What a day!

Yes, in the end we made it to the end, and I was very happy to see my father with his fist medal around his neck.

Glucose-wise, I am happy with my management during the race. I woke up early to have a protein breakfast and planned to eat bit by bit during the ride. Despite being conservative with eating, my glucose levels rose due to the adrenaline of the race.

After 50 km, we made a brief stop where I injected 1 unit of insulin to lower my glucose, which was consistently at 250 mg/dL. Finally, my glucose dropped just in time for the end of the race, allowing me to eat two protein bars during the last 50 km.

In addition to the Dam to Dam, I participated in several other races such as the Amstel Gold Race and Gran Fondo Rosa, Rapha Women 100 Kilometers. During the spring and summer of 2023, I had ridden more than 5000 kilometers.

AMSTERDAM MARATHON 8 KM

Coming back from the Italian summer to the cold and rainy Nether-lands was tough in many ways. Leaving my family behind, the good weather and the holiday feeling made it difficult for me to come back to my daily routine. During the summer, the warm weather helps me stay active while craving less food, causing a reduction of the insulin units I inject. As soon as I reduce the insulin circulating in my body I feel like a new person. I start feeling more energetic in the afterno-on where usually I crash, I have less trouble sleeping and my constant hunger gets reduced. October, November, December, January, and February are challenging months where I need to change my routine to face the winter. Despite the cold and darkness of these months, hol-ding me back from training outside, I had a sport event I really cared about: The Amsterdam Marathon 8-kilometer run! I hadn't partici-pated in a running competition since my knee injury in 2016, so being part of such a big event again was wonderful!

The day finally arrived—a beautiful, sunny Sunday morning. Star-ting from the evening before, I didn't use any carb load strategy as the run was not particularly long for my usual training load. Waking up, my glucose was 150 mg/dL (8.3 mmoL/L). perfect start of the day, I thought. My breakfast was carefully planned and prepared the night before and given the starting glucose I decided not to inject any insulin with my breakfast. I got ready to go, reached the location by bike and started running right away for 8 kilometers. The glucose rose and did not drop below 200 mg/dL (11.1 mmoL/L) for the entire race, and it even rose up to 300 mg/dl (16 mmoL/L). I ran the entire time with a fellow ATAC friend, at 5:30 pace. After the race,

I finally had some food with a normal amount of insulin using my normal carbohydrates to insulin ratio. Unexpectedly high glucose levels occurred and persisted in the evening, probably linked with some adrenaline and cortisol release.

Running burns a lot of sugar, so I was quite scared of hypoglycemia events. In my experience, if the glucose drops too fast it might be impossible to recover in time to perform. After correcting with fast sugar hypoglycemia events, it usually takes 10-15 minutes for the glucose to rise. On the other hand, the adrenaline of the race is always something to consider, playing a role in increasing glucose levels. In my case, the glucose did not drop at all during the exercise as I was running between Zone 3 (Tempo) and Zone 4 (Threshold).

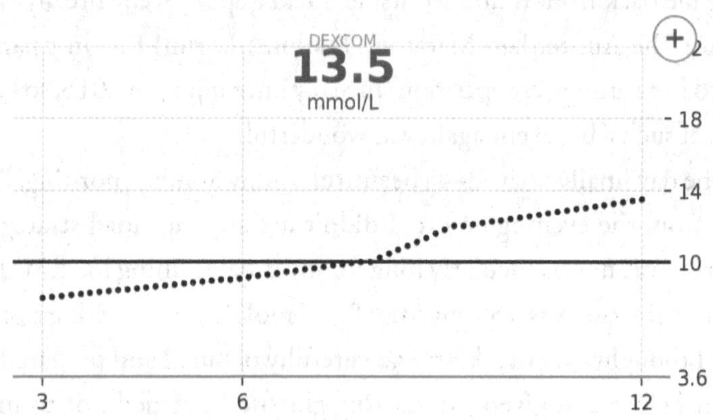

Glucose spiked to 300 mg/dL (14.4 mmoL/L) during the 8k Amsterdam Marathon competition, likely due to adrenaline.

The happiness I felt during the run was overwhelming, and I found myself smiling without a reason. Actually, I knew the reason: The amazing atmosphere. It seemed like a huge street party. There were not only my ATAC friends running with me and cheering on the side but also people from every nationality and age supporting the runners. A group of Swiss grandmas with bells and flags were encouraging the runners, Brazilian groups singing and playing drums and someone dressed up like a lion shouting my name "Go Eleonora!". The most moving thing for me was to notice other athletes with Freestyle Libre and Dexcom CGM running not only as hard, but as happy and proud as I was.

HALF IRONMAN 70.3

Amidst my wavering thoughts, I took the plunge and committed to the 70.3 Ironman in Cervia. Admittedly, I wasn't in peak form, having battled three weeks of antibiotics. Expectations were low, and my primary aim was to enjoy a swim and bike ride, maybe squeezing in a run. But my restless spirit wouldn't let me settle for less, especially on a course devoid of traffic lights and lined with people offering food and drinks.

Imagine Italy at midday, soaking up the hot sun - not your typical setting for a 70.3 race. The event got off to a rocky start when the swim began 45 minutes late due to an object in the water. While 2,540 athletes waited on the beach, the sun continued to beat down. I was glad I didn't decide to wear a wetsuit. The ground we stood on was extremely hot, jumping in the water was soon becoming a necessity.

With the temperature rising and not a single cloud in the sky, finally the race started.

The 2 kilometers swim was less enjoyable than I thought as the sea was too warm, wavy, and full of jellyfish. I finished the swim in a scorching 30 degrees Celsius. Quickly, I hurried to the transition area, checked my glucose, and injected 2 units of Fiasp insulin and 14 units of Tresiba. I decided to delay injecting insulin while swimming for safety reasons.

Once I began biking, I focused on staying hydrated by drinking one water bottle and one electrolyte bottle every 40 kilometers. I ate a whole banana at the 40 kilometers mark while integrating with gels every 40 minutes to keep my energy up.

My glucose levels did not drop for 90 kilometers, but I followed my nutritionist's advice to not panic and not correct it. As predicted, it eventually came down, affecting my legs but also boosting my adrenaline. The last 20 kilometers were extremely difficult due to the strong wind, causing me to feel pain in every part of my body.

Even though my blood sugar levels were still high, I didn't lose hope as I started running. I had a bite of energy bar, hoping it would help bring my energy back up. When I reached the 10-kilometer mark, I started feeling dizzy. My blood sugar dropped rapidly from 300 mg/dL to 150 mg/dL within minutes. I did not feel my glucose dropping, probably because of excitement or tiredness. Now I was in uncharted territory. I had never practiced the full distance. I had never practiced even half of the distance at this time of the day, late afternoon and it never happened to me not to manage to feel a low glucose event.

I did not know if my readings were accurate because of the intense effort I was putting in, I was panicking, I could not breathe, I sat down on the floor.

Calling for assistance, consuming a lot of sugar, gels, and bars while staring at people running like machines. When I realized I was running out of time to finish the race, I pushed myself to go another 2 kilometers. In the end, I had to make the difficult decision to quit, right near the finish line. After enduring 8 grueling hours of competition, I learned that managing diabetes is a huge challenge, much harder than I had ever thought. This 70.3 IRONMAN race turned into an intense battle against diabetes, a life-changing experience. Now, I'm not sure if I can ever be just like everyone else, but one thing is certain - I will never stop trying.

MEAL	INSULIN UNITS	NUTRITION
BREAKFAST	-	3 EGGS 50G BREAD
INTEGRATION 1	2	1 BANANA
INTEGRATION 2	-	1 PROTEIN BAR
INTEGRATION 3	-	1 SIS GEL
INTEGRATION 4	-	

The table shows the number of insulin injections during the half Ironman race day, with the amount (units) and nutrition details.

AMSTERDAM HALF MARATHON

The Amsterdam Half Marathon (21 kilometers) took place on the 14th of October 2023, starting and finishing in the Amsterdam Olympic Stadium. It was a cold, rainy morning that developed into a windy afternoon with some sunny moments alternating with heavy rain. The race started at 1:00 pm, which I really disliked for my diabetes management, as I never go running at 13:00 pm, therefore I have never practiced my glucose and insulin management at that time. It was a difficult start, I decided to have a normal breakfast and a smaller early lunch, not to have an active insulin in the body. During races, I never want to have active insulin (bolus of rapid insulin) as it makes glucose management more difficult, possibly causing fast drops and serious hypoglycemia events.

That morning, I had a normal breakfast and lunch, without excessive carbohydrates. I injected one unit of insulin for breakfast and 2 units for lunch.

- **Breakfast:** 30 grams bread with ham and cheese (20 grams each).
- **Lunch:** Protein bar and a slice of bread with 2 spoons of hummus and 100 grams of roasted vegetables.

To reach the starting point I had to bike a couple of kilometers in the cold, unexpectedly my glucose dropped. My sudden reaction was to integrate with sugar and honey, more than usual as I was about to start running my first half marathon.

As I thought I had everything under control, my glucose started rising due to the adrenaline and cortisol hormones because of the race environment, as soon as I started running. I began the race with elevated glucose, which started dropping after 7 kilometers, causing me some discomfort. I felt lightheaded and panicked, probably more than I should have, given my previous experience with the 70.3 Ironman.

I was carrying a banana and three protein bars with me. I was not carrying additional sugars or extra bananas as I relied on the aid stations for bananas, but by the end of the race, everything was finished. What a horrible situation I was living in. Despite the shortage of water and food at the aid station I managed to keep going.

After this race, I learned an important lesson, always be prepared to rely only on myself. Of course, cause of panic I had too much food and two kilometers before the end, I had to stop and inject some insulin as my glucose was too high, causing discomfort such as a headache and lactic acid in my legs, with glucose levels at 350 mg/dL (17 mmoL/L). After races, I always have trouble lowering my glucose levels due to high stress and adrenaline release. My advice is to be patient and avoid over-correcting with insulin.

The run itself was quite slow, it took me two hours to complete the half marathon, as I was still recovering from four weeks of antibiotics to get rid of E.Coli infection. My heart rate was too high (Zone 4) to push harder, so I made the safe decision to enjoy the day and try again on another race next year.

MALLORCA 2023

From the 26th of March to the 2nd of April 2023, I, along with other members of ATAC, went to Mallorca. This was a completely new experience for me from start to finish, where I had to be mentally flexible with my insulin planning, prepared for any type of technical incident while being able to perform physically.

The triathlon camp was focused on cycling. As a start, I am not a good cycling, in fact I bought my first bike 6 months before Mallorca. Secondly, I had never biked every day for six consecutive days, nor had I experienced high-intensity training for a full week.

Together with my physical challenged, I encountered a couple of unexpected technical failures:

First, my Freestyle Libre (CGM) went out of order after two days, instead of fifteen, because of the heat. Forcing me to replace the CGM in the middle of a bike ride.

Most of the time the CGM data were not accurate, causing the heat, sweat and high effort, misleading me from taking the right decision. On top of that, the data was not available for long periods during the day, as my glucose levels were changing very fast during the bike rides. This caused me extra stress and made this experience even more challenging.

The Freestyle Libre was unreliable on the data, malfunctioning on the transmission, consequently I was unable to check my glucose for long periods. Fortunately, I brought my old-style machine for glucose measurement through finger pricks. This was an important lesson to learn for my diabetes management.

Additionally, to complicate matters, I discovered that my insulin had expired a couple of months earlier, which might have caused erratic insulin behavior. This was totally my fault!

The Mallorca trip was an exhausting trip physically and mentally, my lack of experience combined with the unlucky issues with the Freestyle Libre, made it a big challenge for me. Oh well, I don't like easy things anyway!

Now, back to the fun part. The typical Mallorca camp day was structured as follows: Swim, Bike, Run and Sauna!

The swimming session started in the early morning (7:00 am to 8:00 am). The swimming sessions were self-coached. As Swim director of ATAC I have created swimming training with a different focus for each morning of the week.

After a fresh splash, time for a big buffet breakfast, and then a long bike ride, usually lasting the whole day. The hills were tough to climb but what an amazing view at the top.

Do you still have legs after the ride? Then a running group is waiting for you! Undeniable breathtaking trail running routes and unforgettable sunset runs along the beach, if you had the energy for it.

This was an insane number of activities for my body and most of all for my diabetes management.

One of the challenges for my diabetes management was the breakfast and dinner buffet-style. At first, I thought it was great, but it ended up being even more challenging for me.

I found it hard to perfectly control what I was eating, easily exceeding in carbohydrates and fat. The group pressure of eating a lot to perform and sustain long bike rides dragged me into eating more than I should have, based on the insulin I have injected.

The morning challenge, after engaging my will power for controlling my eating, was to time the insulin perfectly. This is key for a good performance. Despite the departed time being scheduled, most of the time the departing cycling time was delayed causing hyperglycemia.

A second challenge was the increased insulin amount as my breakfast was composed of more carbohydrates than usual. I had to consider that I would have had some active insulin during the rides, creating tiredness and possible hypoglycemia forcing me to stop.

The main goal was to avoid low glucose episodes. In order to do so, I decided to stay on the high side to be safe.

First day, Monday: I had a bigger breakfast than usual, and I managed to count the carbohydrates perfectly. The bike ride was around

60 km on the flat, an easy day to start. I injected two units of insulin, and I took off with the group. Such a success! No need for integration during the ride as I had a protein bar right before the start. In the evening, I felt great, I felt like an hero ready for my next challenge.

Second day, Tuesday: The bike ride was 55 km with two huge climbs in the middle. The ride was high intensity, and the climbs required a higher watt power from my legs, increasing my heart rate to threshold. This situation stressed my body mentally and physically. As a consequence, I faced very high glucose for the next four hours after finishing the bike ride. My body was aching because of the lactic acid I had created during the ride with the impossibility of getting rid of it because of the high glucose.

In order to lower my glucose, I administered four extra units of insulin to bring the glucose back down. Eventually, my glucose came back to normal levels in the afternoon.

Finally at the hotel resting! Oh wait, everyone is going for a run, let me join them! The run was only 3-5 km, but the run was too much for my body.

Thanks to the knowledge I have now I would have avoided the run. Another cardio activity stressed the body even more, creating another spike in glucose. When I got back at the hotel, I was feeling dizzy and very tired.

The third day of cycling, Wednesday: Big day ahead, 90 km bike ride with 800 to 900 meters elevation gain. The morning started early with the usual swim session and carbohydrates combined with protein breakfast.

The day was very hard mentally. The Mallorca group was a strong cycling bunch of people where I was the weakest and least experienced one. Most of the time I was the last one climbing the hills, getting stressed as I was losing the group. Despite the stress, I learned from the experience of the days before to keep the glucose lower in the morning, following the standard insulin to carbohydrate ratio, and having time to integrate during the ride if necessary.

Unfortunately, with diabetes it is impossible to control everything and this time the glucose dropped too fast during the first 30 km of the ride. I immediately integrated with gels that sustained me for the rest of the effort.

The ride had a medium perceived effort till the moment I had to climb. As soon as the hill started and my heart rate increased, as a consequence my glucose spiked up because of the stress hormones. I arrived home pretty tired, my body was hacking for the high glucose and the day after I felt like I was recovering from a cold.

Fourth day, Thursday: I took a rest day with a long swim and a walk along the coast. Overall, a nice and relaxing day! Lesson learned!

The Fifth day, Friday 31st of March, was The Day. The menu had 100 km riding with 1.800 meters elevation gain with steep climbs.

The distance, the elevation gain and the effort were something I had never done before. I was terrified and excited at the same time about how I would have controlled the glucose management during the whole distance, the heat and sustain the constant push on the legs.

That day, I pushed my body and my mind to the limit.

I managed the first climb pretty good; I was satisfied when I stopped for lunch. I have avoided hypoglycemia events and I managed to sustain the effort.

As soon as I stopped for lunch, the carbohydrates from the gels sitting in my stomach kicked off. A glucose spike of 300 mg/dL hit me.

Promptly, I injected 3 units of insulin without eating much.

The glucose spiked down as soon as I started climbing again. This hypoglycemia episode was a very acute and scary one. My eyesight became foggy, my brain obfuscated, and I could not think straight. A friend of mine was ready to spray the glucagon in my nose, but I returned conscious in time.

As soon as I felt better, I kept cycling, leading the group home back to the hotel. Back at the hotel another hypoglycemia event occurred as acute and scary as before, this was the final red flag. My body needed to rest.

The lessons I learned during this holiday were multiple and all of them very important. When injecting insulin during exercise, even if the glucose is high, always consider that the insulin will double or triple its effect, therefore it is important to integrate. The second lesson is to give time to the body to recover, instead of pushing through activities.

Saturday and Sunday were the last two days of the training camp. During the weekend I felt super sensitive to the insulin, the glucose was going up and down very fast, it was impossible for me to understand what was going on in my body. The day was a mix of huge tiredness and frustration for my glucose being uncontrollable.

I decided to enjoy the beauty of Mallorca, going for walks along the beach looking at the sunset. Swimming in the hotel heated outdoor pool was a blast, looking at the blue sky and the palms trees around.

What a unique experience! I am ready to do it all over again next year.

MALLORCA GLUCOSE MANAGEMENT

Departure times varied from 9:30 am to 10:30 am depending on people getting ready, people being late, or last-minute changes. My breakfast was composed of scrambled eggs, with a toasted slice of bread butter with on top ham and cheese. As my breakfast was mainly protein based, I had to eat something to raise my glucose before starting the ride. The breakfast bolus was usually between 2 and 4 units, depending on the starting glucose. The injection time was between 1 hour and 30 minutes to 2 hours before the start of the activity, in order to avoid the insulin peak action while riding. Due to the stress level on my body, I noticed my glucose was reacting very fast to food intake, making it even more challenging to keep it stable.

Breakfast Strategy
- 4 Eggs
- ham and cheese (20 grams each)
- 1 apple before departure.
- 20 grams bread

Biking Strategy

Riding a racing bike can be challenging. Even more challenging is riding a racing bike in a group. The balance on the thin wheels and the group signaling requires focus. There is no time for distraction. In my case I have an extra challenge, diabetes. Checking my glucose constantly, drinking and eating more often than others. While riding at a decent speed I would extract my phone and scan my right arm with the NFC sensor, while carefully balancing my body on the bike. While noticing that my glucose was dropping, a sense of anxiety and sudden fatigue was overwhelming me. I never asked to slow down or take a break because I was ashamed of my own condition, ashamed of my weaknesses.

Most of the time I needed to eat something during the ride, usually every 30 minutes. During a full day biking my integration included one or two SIS gels (which I noticed had a very fast action), two bananas, and protein bars. During these 6 days cycling I had time to test different gels types. My favorite ones were SIS and RioVit. I found that RioVit gels had a longer and steadier action, compared to SIS.

I tried to avoid injecting additional insulin during the ride to prevent low glucose, but on the big ride on Friday, I had to administer additional insulin during the lunch break. The glucose spiked up above 300 mg/dL (16mmL/L) creating lactic acid on my legs and a heavy breathing feeling. Given the situation I decided to inject 1 unit. Frustrated and impatient to perform and feel better as soon as possible I kept checking my glucose value. Only 30 minutes passed, and it seems like 2 hours to me. The glucose was still high (of course), but in an impulsive moment I administered a second unit. Blurred by fatigue and frustration, I grabbed the insulin pen and injected the third unit into my stomach.

Wow! What a roller coaster of emotions and glucose levels. Looking back I would avoid checking in sterically my blood glucose and I would avoid injecting insulin, as the only effect I have obtained was a huge hypoglycemia.

It took me five days to recover and regain my energy, bringing my glucose levels back to stable again. I also had a strong sore throat and a lip herpes outbreak, indicating an immune system deficiency. Overall, it was a great experience as I learned the hard way how to manage my glucose in stressful situations.

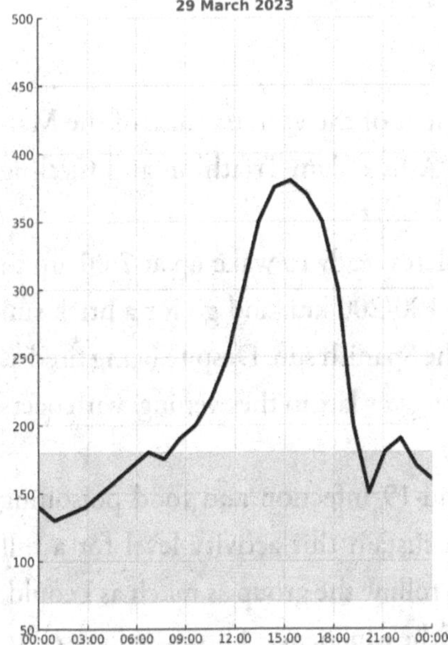

The graph shows my glucose fluctuations during the bike ride on 29th of March and after the ride.

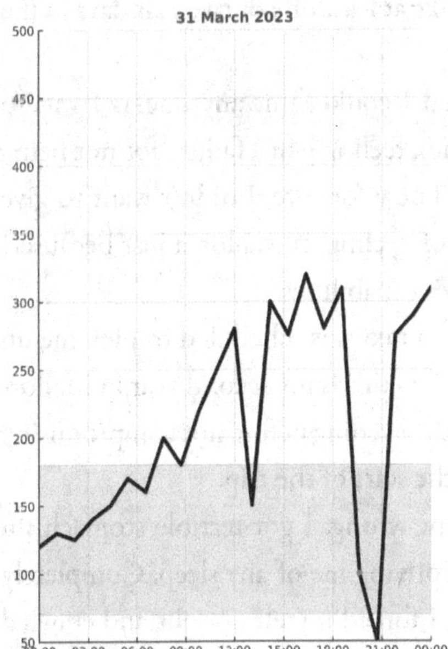

The graph shows my glucose fluctuations during the last day of the Mallorca camp. The body is exhausted.

MALLORCA 2024

April has arrived! The best moment of the year, because of the Mallorca Triathlon Camp with the Amsterdam Triathlon and Cycling Team!

Forty to forty-five excited athletes ready to wake up at 7:00 am to swim couple of kilometers, bike 100-200 km, and go for a brick run afterward: all under the heat of the Spanish sun. Despite being tired at the end of the day, we were ready to stay late in the evening, with beers and wine, chatting and laughing.

Unfortunately, due to a Covid-19 infection and food poisoning the week before, I wasn't fit to sustain this activity level for a full week. Nevertheless, I planned to follow the group as much as I could, enjoying every single moment of the experience. I promised myself to be forgiving with my body and take at least one or two rest days in the middle of the week.

At the beginning, I was scared I could faint anytime as I was so weak. My mind was playing games, feeling like a failure for not being as fit as the others. One thing I knew for sure, I didn't want to give away this amazing opportunity of cycling in Mallorca just because I felt insecure about my own body's capabilities.

On Easter Sunday at 5:00 am, a taxi was scheduled to pick me up and drive me to Schiphol airport. As this is my second year in Mallorca, I carefully planned nutrition the evening before not compromising my energy and glucose level for the start of the trip.

Unfortunately, something went wrong. I got terrible stomach flu that made me vomit all night depriving me of any sleep. Completely dehydrated and without energy, I forced myself upright and crawled down the stairs to meet the taxi. I don't remember anything until another taxi delivered me to the hotel in Mallorca.

This was the start of the holiday. The opposite of what I had planned. The glucose levels were impossible to control, swinging up and down. The body was fighting against sickness and tiredness.

The glucose management was an absolute nightmare! Carefully checking my glucose level every 30 minutes to prevent ketoacidosis. I had constant hyperglycemia, despite not ingesting any food for 48 hours. I was expecting a hypoglycemic episode all the time, as I was regularly injecting insulin, but my glucose stayed solid at 350 mg/dL (above 16 mmoL/L), probably because of the body's stress and inflammation.

I had to spend the following two days in bed, trying to sip water, integrate it with enough electrolytes, and try to keep food inside.

I added an extra handicap on top of managing my diabetes to the Mallorca camp. This was the reality. I felt alone, left behind but finally, on the third day, my energy started increasing.

The sun was shining on my bike that was ready to be used. From Tuesday to Sunday, I managed to bike 60 kilometers every day and swim in the afternoon around 2 kilometers. Unfortunately, I couldn't keep up with the cycling group as the speed and distances were too demanding for my condition, but I had great fun with a few people during shorter rides.

For the entire week I used a consistent nutrition strategy as I was doing similar bike ride distances and intensities. Thanks to the experience I gained the previous year, I managed to have a controlled breakfast composed of around 30 grams of carbohydrates and 30 grams of protein. I was adding fats to my breakfast, such as some butter on toast, flattening the glucose spike curve. I learned to give my body some rest in the afternoon, avoiding overdoing, as I usually tend to do. In this way I managed to have the best time I possibly could during two of my main bike rides, Maria de la Salut and Ca' San Vincent.

MARIA DE LA SALUT

Maria de la Salut bike is an iconic ride in Mallorca! The ride started at 10:00 am, so I had a late breakfast around 9:00 am. Breakfast included 30 grams of cheese, 30 grams of ham and 20 grams of brown bread. The bread acted as a long-lasting carbohydrate, sustaining me during the ride. I added a teaspoon of butter on my toast to add a fat part component, to flatten the sugar spike given by the carbohydrates.

At 8:00 am I injected one unit of insulin, in order not to have the insulin action peak while riding. During the ride, I managed to keep my glucose level stable, integrating with small sip of gels. During the coffee stop in the middle of the ride, I ate half a banana, which caused a slight increase in glucose levels toward the end.

The glucose levels came back in range during the afternoon, when I enjoyed an amazing Aperol Spritz with my fellow ATAC friends by the beach. Another learning day for me and my diabetes. I learned to be more relaxed about my management, forcing myself to not constantly look at my glucose levels but enjoy the beautiful scenery.

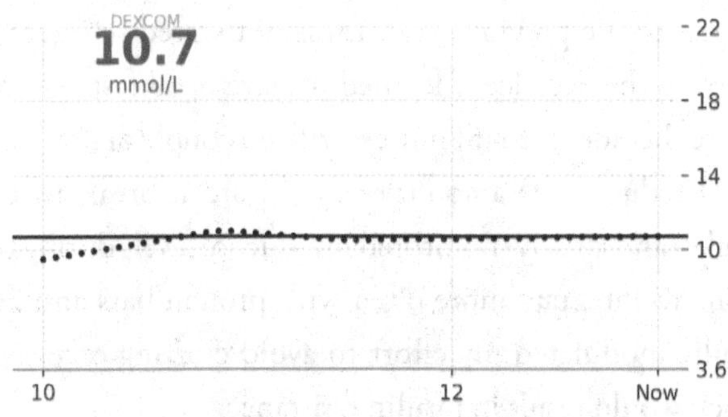

This graph shows that, on average, the blood glucose level during the ride was between 10 and 12 mmoL/L (180 mg/dL -216 mg/dL) over a period of 6 hours.

CA' SAN VINCENT

Ca' San Vincent ride was on a beautiful, sunny day. We biked toward a little beach hidden behind an idyllic forest. That morning, I woke up naturally, with the light coming thought the curtains. While getting ready for breakfast I was happy and grateful to be in Mallorca!

Here we go again, breakfast buffet! I had a light breakfast around 9:00 am with 20 grams of carbohydrates and 30 grams of protein, along with one unit of insulin. I jumped on my bike around 10:00 am and my perceived effort was 6 out of ten. My glucose levels remained stable during the ride, day by day I was feeling better and stronger. I integrated eating a banana half way, without needing additional insulin, despite the glucose value being around 10 mmoL/L.

Having identified the nutrition and insulin strategy that worked for me, made it possible to enjoy the week without excessive body stress and without experiencing significant high or low glucose episodes.

Compared to the previous year, I was not scared to inject insulin before starting the excerice. I learned to have breakfast two to three hours before the ride, even if I must sacrifice a couple of hours of sleep. Moreover, I reduced the amount of food I ate at breakfast to avoid glucose spikes and closely monitored my glucose levels during the ride, allowing me to integrate more often with protein bars and bananas. I successfully modulated my effort to avoid creating excessive body stress, which would result in insulin resistance.

This year, I identified my limits and worked toward raising the bar without constantly exceeding them.

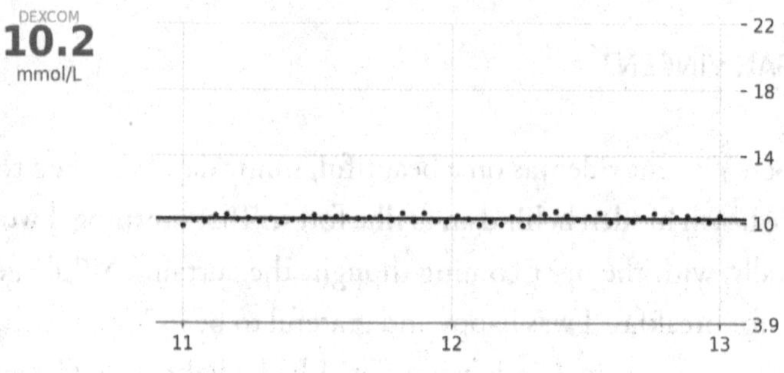

This graph shows that, on average, the blood glucose level was 10 mmoL/L (180 mg/dL) over a period of 6 hours, during and after the bike ride.

I had mixed feelings during this sports holiday—frustration, but also immense gratitude for this great opportunity. I felt fortunate to be healthy enough to bike, enjoy the sun, and savor good food!

Most of the time, I live thinking about what I will do tomorrow, my next goal, or what I will achieve by the end of the year. I often forget to live in the present, catching myself remembering memories.

What I bring home from this experience is a wish for myself: to breathe in the present and enjoy the surprises of life. I love surprises and the adrenaline spike they give me—the unknown feeling. I promised myself to take problems as challenges, or simply as unexpected surprises, but still, surprises!

19. NAVIGATING THE UNEXPECTED

Diabetes is a full-time challenge, but with the right mindset and lifestyle, it can be managed effectively. My mission is to provide genuine insights and practical guidance to those living with diabetes, enhance understanding, and promote a healthy lifestyle.

By sharing my personal experiences, strategies, and the tools I've developed, I aim to inspire others to take control of their health. Combining cognitive behavioral therapies with medical treatments, my goal is to shift the focus from just insulin doses and glucose levels to a comprehensive approach that includes nutrition, exercise, and mental wellbeing. Together, we can create a supportive community where everyone can thrive despite the challenges of diabetes.

Recently, I started a self-discovery process that made me capable of breaking big problems down in small steps, focusing on the small positive accomplishments. Now, as a certified life coach I would like to share what I learned.

ACKNOWLEDGE THE PROBLEM

Acceptance is key! Recognizing and accepting that there is a problem is the first step I take. Seems easy but it's not. Most of the time we make excuses with ourselves, we believe in these excuses that the problem does not actually exist or will disappear and someone else will handle it. It is not the case; you are the author of your own story! Denial could only delay solutions and slow down your path of success towards overcoming the challenge. But first keep calm and focus on the positive.

I learned for myself that practicing mindfulness to stay calm and centered is important. I have not always practiced mindfulness, on the contrary, I wrongly thought it would be not that effective. I considered it a waste of time. Nothing is going to happen if I stay still, right?

Well, in this society where everything moves so fast, practicing slowing down actually helps us to reconnect with our inner self. What helps me in concrete, is to practice Yin Yoga or Yoga Nidra to deeply relax! This really improved my mental health. Surprisingly, I notice positive feedback on my glucose levels as well! Reconnect with your deeper self, as you, and you only have all the answers!

THE PROBLEM IDENTIFICATION

Many times, in my life, something was not going as planned. The sense of frustration was all over my body till the moment I could clearly define the problem. When the issue was too complex, I managed to break it down into smaller, manageable. I noticed that most of the time, talking about the problem will make it seem less dramatic and smaller compared to the original image in my mind. Talking about it will initiate a chain of thought to start looking for solutions.

SET CLEAR GOALS

In my daily job I apply my project management skills to pharmaceutical companies. Working in a goal orientated environment helped me to learn how to create SMART goals. Nothing too hard, don't worry! Set Specific, Measurable, Achievable, Relevant, and Time-bound goals to address the problem! This process will help create clarity in your mind and naturally prioritize what is more urgent to resolve.

Now is the moment to implement your plan with confidence! Take decisive action rather than procrastinating! The moment to act is now! Perhaps starting with practicing self-care. Here are some examples of what I do.

- *Practicing Yin Yoga* twice a week helped me reduce body and mind stress levels. Moreover, I notice lower glucose values during the two hours post meditation.
- *Beauty care* once a week, such as applying a face mask, or take a long hot bath helps me distend my nerves and lose muscular tension.
- *Practice Sport every day!* I cannot imagine my life without it! It is not only beneficial for improving my glucose levels, but it gives me energy to carry on other boring daily tasks.

By following these steps, you can systematically and effectively address problems, turning challenges into opportunities for growth and improvement.

My conclusion is that bad days are always around the corner, but they are flattened by the volume of good days that we get in, if we live intentionally and we set clear priorities.

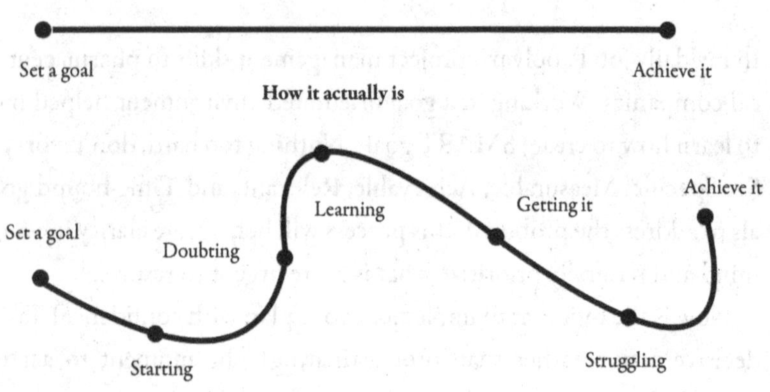

The figure shows the path of setting goals: expectations vs. reality. That's why reality is so much more fun!

THE CHALLENGES OF A NEW ROUTINE

Initiating a new routine can be an arduous task, often fraught with numerous obstacles and challenges. Whether it's logging food intake, documenting physical activities, or tracking glucose levels, the initial phase of establishing these habits demands a significant amount of effort, consistency, and dedication. However, despite the inherent difficulties, the benefits of maintaining such routines can be profoundly rewarding, offering enhanced health outcomes, better disease management, and an overall improved quality of life.

One of the primary challenges I experienced is the sheer volume of data that needs to be recorded. Every meal, snack, and beverage must be logged meticulously, carbohydrate content, portion sizes, and timing.

Similarly, each bout of physical activity, including its duration, intensity, and type, must be documented. The task can seem daunting, especially for those like me, who are not accustomed to such detailed record-keeping.

In addition to the practical challenges, there are significant psychological barriers to overcome. The idea of committing to a new routine can be intimidating, often leading to procrastination or abandonment of the effort altogether. It requires a shift in mindset, from viewing the routine as a chore to seeing it as an integral part of daily life. This mental adjustment was crucial in my path but was quite difficult to achieve.

Motivation plays a key role in overcoming these barriers. The initial enthusiasm wanes quickly, especially when results are not immediately visible. It is easy to become disheartened and question the value of the effort, particularly when faced with the daily demands of life, work, and other responsibilities.

Despite the initial difficulties, persistence pays off. Gradually, what was once a challenging task becomes a habit. The process of logging food and exercise becomes more intuitive and less time-consuming. What happened to me was that the patterns in glucose levels became clearer, allowing better diabetes management.

I started and stopped the food and sport logging routine multiple times before it became a habit. The key is to start small and build gradually. Begin with logging one meal a day or tracking exercise for a few minutes each session. As these smaller tasks become routine, it becomes easier to expand the scope. Setting achievable goals and celebrating small victories can help maintain motivation and build confidence.

Moreover, the routine itself can foster a greater sense of control and empowerment. Knowing that you are taking proactive steps to manage your health can boost confidence and reduce anxiety. The data collected over time provides valuable insights, allowing for more informed decisions and adjustments to the management plan. Give it a go yourself now!

MEAL	TIME	OPTION 1	OPTION 2	OPTION 3
BREAKFAST				
SNACK				
LUNCH				
SNACK				
DINNER				
SNACK				

The table serves as a structured guide for organizing meals and snacks throughout the week.

DATE	MORNING	LUNCH	BEFORE DINNER	AFTER DINNER
MONDAY				
TUESDAY				
WEDNESDAY				
THURSDAY				
FRIDAY				
SATURDAY				
SUNDAY				

The table is a structural guide to organize your training.

20. DIABETES FOR ALL

My father never deeply understood the real effort I was putting into planning and structuring my daily sport and nutrition, until the day he read this diary. I was really surprised by his reaction. I was assuming that parents know their kids inside out. I was assuming that there is no need to explain how I felt, but I was wrong. I had the wrong image of my dad being a super dad. Unfortunately, not, and with time I released him and I should not know everything either. My father admitted that he never realized what was behind each of my decisions. He was surprised to read the reasoning behind my requests to stop and take a break while biking. He told me it was very hard to imagine such a complicated and structured plan behind every run or swim training.

This fact made me realize that it is hard for a parent to fully understand what's going on in the head of their kids. I have had Diabetes since 1999, I was three years old and at the time it was easy for my parents, as I was not making any decisions. During my teenagers' years everything changed. I took control of my diabetes and most of the time I would tell my parents "All good, everything is fine".

Most of all, what was underestimated by many doctors, including my father who is one, is the psychological impact of diabetes, that is not solvable with additional medication but only with sharing the difficulties, listening carefully, loving unconditionally and compassion.

Before leaving to Amsterdam, I asked for help in many ways, many times from my family but felt like I was left alone.

I now understand that perhaps my requests for help were not understood or not clearly expressed. This diary could be a help for parents to understand deeply what is going on behind the scenes, in the heads of their kids, providing not only practical help for people with diabetes but also emotional support and understanding.

Dear parents, I am not sure how much you should check on your son or daughter, how much you should ask how they are doing, or ask what their glucose value is, but one thing I can tell you, trust them, because they are incredibly strong!

THE RIPPLE EFFECT OF DIABETES

The psychological impact of diabetes is a topic close to my heart. During my almost 30 years with diabetes, I don't remember anyone explaining the psychological impact of this chronic disease, without a cure. Unfortunately, my hospital did not provide emotional support for me or my family to guide us through the possible feelings that could come my way during my diabetes journey. The following paragraphs are the diabetes truth, something everyone, whether they have diabetes or not, should be aware of.

Diabetes is a condition that extends its influence beyond the individual who lives with it. It touches the lives of family members and partners, and the journey involves unique challenges and shared responsibilities. The most difficult part of diabetes comes when we need to share our feelings, which most of the time are a deep sense of frustration and failure. Understanding this ripple effect and fostering open communication can help alleviate the emotional burden and strengthen the support network around those living with diabetes.

I have had diabetes since I was three years old, and I do not know how my life without it would be. Some of us are naturally more reserved and may find it difficult to openly discuss diabetes, especially with family, friends, or life companions. The anxiety of revealing this aspect of our lives can be daunting, and we often anticipate the same recurring questions from those around us where we use the same answers. "Yes, I can eat everything". We repeat this mantra, striving to blend in, but the reality is more complex. There are times when sugar is a no-go, but there are also instances where we desperately need it, and we need it fast. Unfortunately, there's the daily routine of finger pricks, insulin injections, or being tethered to an insulin pump, which, let's face it, isn't the coolest thing. All I desire is to be just like everyone else, to be as effortlessly cool as the most popular girl in school, who, of course, doesn't have diabetes. Having friends was hard during elementary school where I remember I was feeling different in some ways. Afterwards, becoming a teenager was also challenging and I had to be more controlling and less spontaneous compared to my friends.

The social media era began; everything is out there to be shown; our houses, our friends, our habits, and our bodies. My life with diabetes suddenly looked less nice. Affected by diabetes and hypothyroidism, losing weight can be a struggle, and gaining weight can feel all too easy, especially around the injection sites. This is the insulin effect itself, creating adipose tissue and promoting the feeling of hunger.

Here's the thing I am sharing as a girl who has been a teenager with diabetes: if the average girl may struggle with eating disorders and panic attacks related to body weight, imagine what it's like for a diabetic girl. I know girls who fear the idea of being on a diet or counting calories. Unfortunately, I was one of them myself, although, with diabetes

I need to do that. I need to count every gram of carbohydrates, protein and fat in my plate in order to achieve the perfect management. The burden of diabetes is underestimated, and I am asking myself why aren't we talking more about this? Why don't we have more psychological support?

The psychological impact of diabetes can be profound and multifaceted, affecting individuals in various ways:

- **Emotional Distress:** A diabetes diagnosis can lead to a range of emotional responses, including shock, sadness, anger, and anxiety. Coping with the daily demands of managing the condition, such as blood sugar monitoring, insulin injections, or medication, can be emotionally taxing.

- **Stress and Burnout:** The constant vigilance required for diabetes management can lead to chronic stress and, in some cases, diabetes burnout. Burnout is characterized by feelings of frustration, exhaustion, and a desire to temporarily disengage from self-care responsibilities.

- **Depression:** Research has shown that people with diabetes are at a higher risk of developing depression. The stress of managing the condition, concerns about potential complications, and the impact on daily life can contribute to depressive symptoms.

- **Anxiety:** The fear of hypoglycemia, hyperglycemia, or diabetes-related complications can lead to anxiety. I worry everyday about the future and the unpredictability of this condition.

- **Body Image and Self-Esteem:** Changes in body weight or shape, especially when starting insulin treatment, can impact body image and self-esteem. This is particularly true in my life as it was never easy to accept my body. The frustration I get is unexplainable, because despite the diet and exercise plan I follow, I do not achieve the same results as my fellow athletes' friends.

- **Social and Relationship Challenges:** Diabetes can affect relationships, as family members may worry about the person with diabetes, and managing the condition can sometimes disrupt social activities.
- **Stigma and Discrimination:** Some individuals may encounter stigma or discrimination related to their diabetes. This can lead to feelings of unfairness, frustration, or isolation.
- **Diabetes Distress:** Diabetes-specific distress is a unique form of psychological distress related to the condition. It includes feelings of guilt, fear, and frustration about living with diabetes and its management.

During these 30 years with diabetes, I have developed various coping strategies to manage the psychological impact. These can be positive, such as engaging in support groups or exercise, or negative, such as avoidance behaviors or unhealthy eating habits. The psychological impact at times influenced my adherence to treatment plans. In a period of my life I struggled with self-care tasks, such as taking medication, monitoring blood sugar, or maintaining a healthy lifestyle.

I was lost. One day, I was walking in nature, and I remember a prayer my mum told me once.

A woman was walking in the desert for days. Tired and hungry, without hope anymore. Hallucinations started coming though her head and she lost consciousness. She woke up traumatized and upset. The woman was staring at the dunes, and she could see the footprints left on the send. Right foot, left foot, right foot, left foot.

The woman started complaining to God, why did you do this to me? Why did you abandon me here? A voice replied to her: "I never abandoned you; When you fell, I carried you on my shoulder."

A spark in my head made me realize that I will never be alone, but I need to be the first one to take care of myself no matter what, no matter the difficulties. I know that light is guiding me towards my goal, and I can feel a hand on my shoulder reassuring me every day.

PSYCHOLOGICAL SUPPORT

I have always battled through diabetes distress, depression, and anxiety. It is important to acknowledge the psychological aspect of diabetes and to tell everyone not to be ashamed to seek support when needed. I hope this chapter raises awareness about this crucial issue.

I am deeply grateful to my family for always being supportive and embarking on the learning journey of diabetes with me since 1999. Their unconditional support has been invaluable. In addition to my family's support, I have finally found a life companion with whom I can be myself, without the need to hide the moments of frustration that people with diabetes experience. Having someone, like my boyfriend, supportive in all the small day-to-day things—making sure the eating time is good for me and that there is the right food on the table depending on my glucose levels—is fundamental for less stressful diabetes management. These little things are essential for a smoother journey with diabetes alongside your family and partner.

DIABETES WITH MY FAMILY

My family played a crucial role in understanding the nuances of diabetes, learning about blood sugar monitoring, insulin injections, dietary requirements, and the signs of hypo- and hyperglycemia. It was a big shock for us all in 1999, and it meant lifestyle changes for the whole family. At the time, technology was poor, so I had to learn how to cut my fingers and inject insulin at the age of three. My mom had been leaving me at school since 8:00 am and there were no remote controls to check the glucose of the kids as today. A big shoutout for my mom that was controlling without being controlling, she was preoccupied without making me feel she was preoccupied. She was trusting me, and I felt the trust! During the years I was living at home, my family shifted the meal planning towards healthier options, and exercise became a family affair. There was increased vigilance about managing stress and overall well-being all through my childhood. I remember with much happiness the bike ride on a Sunday, the roller skating in the park and the walks along the river.

Last but not least, I had great emotional support from my grandparents, as diabetes can be emotionally taxing. Everyone witnessed me facing stress, anxiety, and even depression. Providing emotional support and being mindful of these challenges was, and still is, essential for me. Being united as a family in making lifestyle changes is key to succeeding in the goals.

DIABETES WITH MY PARTNER

Matthew and I met in 2018, in Amsterdam. At the time, he was a marketing master student at the same university where I was completing my Oncology master's degree, Matt was love at first sight. Now Matt is not only my life partner, but he is an active participant in my life with diabetes. He shares the responsibility of maintaining a diabetes-friendly home environment, often taking on the task of meal planning and preparation and ensuring that healthy options are readily available. He even adapts recipes to accommodate my dietary restrictions, adding less sugar, minimizing the carbohydrates, avoiding the fats. Now, Matt is used to homemade banana bread and chocolate cakes with less than 50 grams of sugar inside, he is used to taking sorbetto instead of gelato, and making everything possible to decrease my chances of glucose spikes. He supports me every day with small gestures such as when he decided to walk with me, after dinner in the cold and rainy Amsterdam. Matt is used to a protein-based diet and now he likes eggs for dinner, which he was only considering as a breakfast meal.

Managing diabetes can be an emotional rollercoaster, and Matt offers unwavering emotional support. He is there to listen, provide reassurance, and help me cope with challenges.

What I have experienced is a journey that involves adapting to a new way of life, marked by understanding, compassion, and teamwork. Diabetes isn't just an individual's condition; it's a shared experience, and the support and active involvement of family and partners play a pivotal role in ensuring a thriving and fulfilling life despite the challenges.

21. CONCLUSIONS

Reflecting on my journey with type 1 diabetes, I am filled with profound gratitude and a sense of accomplishment. Managing this condition as an athlete has been a formidable challenge, requiring constant vigilance, dedication, and adaptability. From the early days of my diagnosis to my current endeavors as an athlete and advocate, each step has been marked by both struggles and triumphs.

"The focus on Nutrition and Sport" has been pivotal in my approach to diabetes management. One of the most significant lessons I've learned is the importance of a holistic approach to diabetes care. This journey has underscored the critical role of nutrition, exercise, and emotional well-being in maintaining stable glucose levels and overall health. Adopting a low-carbohydrate diet, not as a restrictive regimen but as a mindful method of eating, has transformed my life. By carefully planning meals and focusing on reducing glucose spikes, I have minimized the need for excessive insulin and achieved greater glucose stability.

Physical activity has also been a cornerstone of my diabetes management. Engaging in various forms of exercise, from swimming and biking to running, has not only improved my physical health but also provided emotional and psychological benefits. Training in lower heart rate zones, optimizing fat oxidation, and carefully monitoring glucose levels with food integration during workouts have been key strategies in managing my condition effectively during sport.

The emotional aspect of living with diabetes cannot be overstated. Battling diabetes distress, depression, and anxiety has been an integral part of my experience. I have come to understand the value of seeking psychological support and the importance of a strong support network. My family's and my partner's active involvement have been invaluable in navigating the complexities of this condition.

Through this journey, I have also learned the importance of education and awareness. Understanding the historical context of diabetes management and the evolution of treatment approaches has provided valuable insights into the current challenges and opportunities for improvement. It is crucial for healthcare professionals, patients, and their families to stay informed and embrace a proactive approach to diabetes care.

In conclusion, my experience with type 1 diabetes has been a journey of continuous learning and growth. It has taught me resilience, patience, and the power of a positive mindset. While the road has been challenging, it has also been filled with moments of joy, achievement, and deep connection with those who support me. I hope that my experiences and insights can serve as a source of inspiration and guidance for others navigating their own diabetes journey. Together, we can strive for a healthier, more fulfilling life, embracing each challenge as an opportunity for growth.

ACKNOWLEDGMENT

I would like to express my heartfelt gratitude to a multitude of individuals who have played a significant role in my journey. First and foremost, my family deserves a monumental thank you. To my mother, my unwavering rock of support, Alessandra is more than a mother, she is my best friend and my angel. To my father, I owe an immeasurable gratitude, for pushing me above my limits, supporting my challenges. My sister, the keeper of my heart, also holds a special place in this acknowledgment. Federica is not only my sister, she is the reason why I feel complete and safe in this world, knowing that she will always be by my side. A big thank you to my aunts Paola and Silvia, who represent the symbols of strong women for me, inspiring me during my journey.

In my time in Turin, Italy, I encountered a remarkable team of medical professionals, and I must extend my thanks to them. Dott. Saccheti, Dott. Cerutti, Dott.Grassi and the nurses Patrizia and Rosaria were instrumental in my care. Additionally, I am immensely appreciative of the guidance and care provided by Dott. Rabbone, Dott. Gallone, Dott. Gaita, Dott. Aranzulla and many others who crossed my path during my medical journey in Turin.

My fitness and wellness journey would not have been the same without the invaluable contributions of my Italian gym and spinning instructors, Teresa, Francesca, Davide, Marco, and Celeste. My swim instructor, Cesare, also deserves my gratitude as my sparks for competitions started with him at the Master Swimming Team at San

Giuseppe School. San Giuseppe has a special place in my heart, mostly because of the guidance, teaching, and life support from Prof. R. Barbero. Above all, I want to acknowledge the profound impact the Amsterdam Triathlon and Cycling club, in the Netherlands, had on reshaping my approach to training. I'm deeply grateful to my triathlon and non-triathlon friends accompanying me in this journey and to myself for the dedication and determination I had.

I am indebted to several individuals who have been integral to my overall well-being and success. My nutritionist, Wesley, and my personal trainer, Joost, who were a guiding light on this journey. Bas Van der Goor has provided unwavering support and encouragement. Matt, my second personal trainer, and Vincent, Max, Guido and Robin, my physiotherapists, have played pivotal roles in my physical well-being. The staff at Amsterdam, OLGV West hospital, too numerous to name individually, have contributed to my journey in meaningful ways.

Lastly, I must express my deep appreciation to my boyfriend, Matthew, for his unwavering encouragement throughout the ups and downs of this journey. I want to thank him, because he makes me feel at home in the Netherlands and thank him for being my family. Additionally, I want to thank Michiel, the Product Owner of JJT, for inspiring and empowering me to pursue my passions. Most of all, my manager Saskia has been supporting me along this life and career journey from the day we met.

To all these individuals, and to the countless others who have supported me in various ways, I extend my sincerest thanks for being a part of this incredible journey. Your contributions have made a profound difference in my life, and I am forever grateful.

REFERENCES

1. American Diabetes Association. (2020). Standards of Medical Care in Diabetes—2020. Diabetes Care, 43(Supplement 1), S1-S212. https://doi.org/10.2337/dc20-SINT

2. Banting, F. G., Best, C. H., Collip, J. B., Campbell, W. R., & Fletcher, A. A. (1922). Pancreatic extracts in the treatment of diabetes mellitus. Canadian Medical Association Journal, 12(3), 141-146.

3. Basu, R., Dalla Man, C., Campioni, M., Basu, A., Klee, G., Toffolo, G.,& Rizza, R. A. (2009). Mechanisms of postprandial hyperglycemia in elderly men and women: gender-specific differences in insulin secretion and action. Diabetes, 58(3), 699-705. https://doi.org/10.2337/db08-0916

4. Bode, B. W., & Testa, M. A. (1997). Insulin pump therapy: Impact on quality of life and glycemic control. Diabetes Care, 20(3), 364-369. https://doi.org/10.2337/diacare.20.3.364

5. Cantani, A. (1999). The principles and practice of low-carbohydrate living. Journal of Diabetes and Metabolic Disorders, 23(4), 295-308.

6. Caprio, S., Perry, R., & Kursawe, R. (2012). Adolescent obesity and insulin resistance: roles of ectopic fat accumulation and adipose

inflammation. Gastroenterology, 142(6), 1231-1243. https://doi.org/10.1053/j.gastro.2012.04.001

7. Cersosimo, E., & DeFronzo, R. A. (2006). Insulin resistance and endothelial dysfunction: the road map to cardiovascular diseases. Diabetes Metabolism Research and Reviews, 22(6), 423-436. https://doi.org/10.1002/dmrr.634

8. Diabetes Control and Complications Trial Research Group. (1993). The effect of intensive treatment of diabetes on the development and progression of long-term complications in insulin-dependent diabetes mellitus. New England Journal of Medicine, 329(14), 977-986. https://doi.org/10.1056/NEJM199309303291401

9. Dunning, T. (2014). Care of People with Diabetes: A Manual of Nursing Practice. Wiley-Blackwell.

10. Evert, A. B., Dennison, M., Gardner, C. D., Garvey, W. T., Lau, K. H., MacLeod, J.,& Yancy, W. S. (2019). Nutrition therapy for adults with diabetes or prediabetes: a consensus report. Diabetes Care, 42(5), 731-754. https://doi.org/10.2337/dci19-0014

11. Gaede, P., Lund-Andersen, H., Parving, H. H., & Pedersen, O. (2008). Effect of a multifactorial intervention on mortality in type 2 diabetes. New England Journal of Medicine, 358(6), 580-591. https://doi.org/10.1056/NEJMoa0706245

12. Gale, E. A. M., & Gillespie, K. M. (2001). Diabetes and gender. Diabetologia, 44(1), 3-15. https://doi.org/10.1007/s001250051573

13. Gerstein, H. C., Miller, M. E., Byington, R. P., Goff, D. C., Bigger, J. T., Buse, J. B.,& ACCORD Study Group. (2008). Effects of intensive glucose lowering in type 2 diabetes. New England Journal of Medicine, 358(24), 2545-2559. https://doi.org/10.1056/NEJMoa0802743

14. Goldstein, D. E., Little, R. R., Lorenz, R. A., Malone, J. I., Nathan, D., & Peterson, C. M. (2004). Tests of glycemia in diabetes. Diabetes Care, 27(7), 1761-1773. https://doi.org/10.2337/diacare.27.7.1761

15. Gregory, J. W., & Amiel, S. A. (2007). Hypoglycemia in diabetes. Blackwell Publishing.

16. Hirsch, I. B., & Bergenstal, R. M. (2010). Insulin in the treatment of diabetes: a chapter in the history of medicine. In R. A. DeFronzo, F. Ferrannini, P. Zimmet, & K. G. Alberti (Eds.), International Textbook of Diabetes Mellitus (4th ed., pp. 655-672). Wiley-Blackwell.

17. Holman, R. R., Paul, S. K., Bethel, M. A., Matthews, D. R., & Neil, H. A. W. (2008). 10-year follow-up of intensive glucose control in type 2 diabetes. New England Journal of Medicine, 359(15), 1577-1589. https://doi.org/10.1056/NEJMoa0806470

18. Inzucchi, S. E., Bergenstal, R. M., Buse, J. B., Diamant, M., Ferrannini, E., Nauck, M.,& Matthews, D. R. (2012). Management of hyperglycemia in type 2 diabetes: a patient-centered approach: position statement of the American Diabetes Association (ADA) and the European Association for the Study of Diabetes (EASD). Diabetes Care, 35(6), 1364-1379. https://doi.org/10.2337/dc12-0413

19. Kahn, S. E., Haffner, S. M., Heise, M. A., Herman, W. H., Holman, R. R., Jones, N. P.,& Viberti, G. (2006). Glycemic durability of rosiglitazone, metformin, or glyburide monotherapy. New England Journal of Medicine, 355(23), 2427-2443. https://doi.org/10.1056/NEJMoa066224

20. King, P., Peacock, I., & Donnelly, R. (1999). The UK Prospective Diabetes Study (UKPDS): clinical and therapeutic implications for type 2 diabetes. British Journal of Clinical Pharmacology, 48(5), 643-648. https://doi.org/10.1046/j.1365-2125.1999.00092.x

21. Knowler, W. C., Barrett-Connor, E., Fowler, S. E., Hamman, R. F., Lachin, J. M., Walker, E. A., & Nathan, D. M. (2002). Reduction in the incidence of type 2 diabetes with lifestyle intervention or metformin. New England Journal of Medicine, 346(6), 393-403. https://doi.org/10.1056/NEJMoa012512

22. LeRoith, D., Smith, D. O., & Molitch, M. E. (2012). Prevention and treatment of type 2 diabetes: a stepwise approach. Diabetes Care, 35(Supplement 1), S99-S104. https://doi.org/10.2337/dc12-s015

23. Nathan, D. M., Cleary, P. A., Backlund, J. Y. C., Genuth, S. M., Lachin, J. M., Orchard, T. J.,& Diabetes Control and Complications Trial/Epidemiology of Diabetes Interventions and Complications (DCCT/EDIC) Study Research Group. (2005). Intensive diabetes treatment and cardiovascular disease in patients with type 1 diabetes. New England Journal of Medicine, 353(25), 2643-2653. https://doi.org/10.1056/NEJMoa052187

24. Nathan, D. M., Genuth, S., Lachin, J., Cleary, P., Crofford, O., Davis, M.,& Diabetes Control and Complications Trial Research Group. (1993). The effect of intensive treatment of diabetes on the development and progression of long-term complications in insulin-dependent diabetes mellitus. New England Journal of Medicine, 329(14), 977-986. https://doi.org/10.1056/NEJM199309303291401

25. Pories, W. J., Swanson, M. S., MacDonald, K. G., Long, S. B., Morris, P. G., Brown, B. M.,& Barakat, H. A. (1995). Who would have thought it? An operation proves to be the most effective therapy for adult-onset diabetes mellitus. Annals of Surgery, 222(3), 339-350. https://doi.org/10.1097/00000658-199509000-00011

26. Powers, M. A., Bardsley, J. K., Cypress, M., Duker, P., Funnell, M. M., Hess Fischl, A.,& Vivian, E. (2015). Diabetes self-management education and support in type 2 diabetes: a joint position statement of the American Diabetes Association, the American Association of Diabetes Educators, and the Academy of Nutrition and Dietetics. Diabetes Care, 38(7), 1372-1382. https://doi.org/10.2337/dc15-0730

27. Ratner, R. E. (2012). An update on the Diabetes Prevention Program. Endocrine Practice, 18(4), 600-608. https://doi.org/10.4158/EP12151.RA

28. Rubin, R. R., & Peyrot, M. (2001). Psychological issues and treatments for people with diabetes. Journal of Clinical Psychology, 57(4), 457-478. https://doi.org/10.1002/jclp.1041

29. Saydah, S. H., & Lochner, K. A. (2010). Socioeconomic status and risk of diabetes-related mortality in the US. Public Health Reports, 125(3), 377-388. https://doi.org/10.1177/003335491012500308

30. Skyler, J. S., Bergenstal, R., Bonow, R. O., Buse, J., Deedwania, P., Gale, E. A. M.,& Sherwin, R. S. (2009). Intensive glycemic control and the prevention of cardiovascular events: implications of the ACCORD, ADVANCE, and VA diabetes trials: a position statement of the American Diabetes Association and a scientific statement of the American College of Cardiology Foundation and the American Heart Association. Diabetes Care, 32(1), 187-192. https://doi.org/10.2337/dc08-9026

31. Stolar, M. W. (2010). Atherosclerosis in diabetes: the role of hyperinsulinemia. Metabolism, 59(Supplement 1), S1-S3. https://doi.org/10.1016/j.metabol.2010.07.003

32. Stratton, I. M., Adler, A. I., Neil, H. A., Matthews, D. R., Manley, S. E., Cull, C. A.,& Holman, R. R. (2000). Association of glycaemia with macrovascular and microvascular complications of

type 2 diabetes (UKPDS 35): prospective observational study. BMJ, 321(7258), 405-412. https://doi.org/10.1136/bmj.321.7258.405

33. Taubes, G. (2008). Good calories, bad calories: Fats, carbs, and the controversial science of diet and health. Anchor Books.

34. Tuomilehto, J., Lindström, J., Eriksson, J. G., Valle, T. T., Hämäläinen, H., Ilanne-Parikka, P.,& Uusitupa, M. (2001). Prevention of type 2 diabetes mellitus by changes in lifestyle among subjects with impaired glucose tolerance. New England Journal of Medicine, 344(18), 1343-1350. https://doi.org/10.1056/NEJM200105033441801

35. Turner, R. C., Millns, H., Neil, H. A., Stratton, I. M., Manley, S. E., Matthews, D. R., & Holman, R. R. (1998). Risk factors for coronary artery disease in non-insulin dependent diabetes mellitus: United Kingdom Prospective Diabetes Study (UKPDS: 23). BMJ, 316(7134), 823-828. https://doi.org/10.1136/bmj.316.7134.823

36. U.K. Prospective Diabetes Study Group. (1998). Intensive blood-glucose control with sulphonylureas or insulin compared with conventional treatment and risk of complications in patients with type 2 diabetes (UKPDS 33). The Lancet, 352(9131), 837-853. https://doi.org/10.1016/S0140-6736(98)07019-6

37. van Dieren, S., Beulens, J. W., van der Schouw, Y. T., Grobbee, D. E., & Neal, B. (2010). The global burden of diabetes and its complications: an emerging pandemic. European Journal of Cardiova-

scular Prevention & Rehabilitation, 17(1_suppl), S3-S8. https://doi.org/10.1097/01.hjr.0000368191.86614.5a

38. Van Gaal, L. F., Mertens, I. L., & De Block, C. E. (2006). Mechanisms linking obesity with cardiovascular disease. Nature, 444(7121), 875-880. https://doi.org/10.1038/nature05487

39. Vijan, S., & Hayward, R. A. (2004). Treatment of hypertension in type 2 diabetes mellitus: blood pressure goals, choice of agents, and setting priorities in diabetes care. Annals of Internal Medicine, 138(7), 593-602.   https://doi.org/10.7326/0003-4819-138-7-200304010-00014

40. Wadden, T. A., Neiberg, R. H., Wing, R. R., Clark, J. M., Delahanty, L. M., Hill, J. O.,& Look AHEAD Research Group. (2011). Four-year weight losses in the Look AHEAD study: factors associated with long-term success. Obesity, 19(10), 1987-1998. https://doi.org/10.1038/oby.2011.230

41. Wild, S., Roglic, G., Green, A., Sicree, R., & King, H. (2004). Global prevalence of diabetes: estimates for the year 2000 and projections for 2030. Diabetes Care, 27(5), 1047-1053. https://doi.org/10.2337/diacare.27.5.1047

42. Wing, R. R., & Goldstein, M. G. (1991). Behavioral strategies in the treatment of obesity. In A. J. Stunkard & T. A. Wadden (Eds.), Obesity: Theory and therapy (2nd ed., pp. 432-444). Raven Press.

43. Wright, L. A., & Hirsch, I. B. (2012). The challenge of the upper limit: the target A1c for type 1 diabetes. Diabetes Care, 35(12), 2468-2475. https://doi.org/10.2337/dc12-0804

44. Yki-Järvinen, H. (2004). Thiazolidinediones. New England Journal of Medicine, 351(11), 1106-1118. https://doi.org/10.1056/NEJMra041001

45. Zimmet, P. Z., Magliano, D. J., Herman, W. H., & Shaw, J. E. (2014). Diabetes: a 21st century challenge. The Lancet Diabetes & Endocrinology, 2(1), 56-64. https://doi.org/10.1016/S2213-8587(13)70112-8

46. Riddell MC, Scott SN, Fournier PA, Colberg SR, Gallen IW, Moser O, Stettler C, Yardley JE, Zaharieva DP, Adolfsson P, Bracken RM. The competitive athlete with type 1 diabetes. Diabetologia. 2020 Aug;63(8):1475-1490. doi: 10.1007/s00125-020-05183-8.

47. Riddell MC, Peters AL. Exercise in adults with type 1 diabetes mellitus. Nat Rev Endocrinol. 2023 Feb;19(2):98-111. doi: 10.1038/s41574-022-00756-6.

48. Riddell MC, Gallen IW, Smart CE, Taplin CE, Adolfsson P, Lumb AN, Kowalski A, Rabasa-Lhoret R, McCrimmon RJ, Hume C, Annan F, Fournier PA, Graham C, Bode B, Galassetti P, Jones TW, Millán IS, Heise T, Peters AL, Petz A, Laffel LM. Exercise management in type 1 diabetes: a consensus statement. Lancet Diabetes Endocrinol. 2017 May;5(5):377-390. doi: 10.1016/S2213-8587(17)30014-1.

49. Riddell MC, Gallen IW, Rabasa-Lhoret R; JDRF-T1D Performance in Exercise and Knowledge Working Group. Exercise and physical activity in patients with type 1 diabetes - Authors' reply. Lancet Diabetes Endocrinol. 2017 Jul;5(7):493-494. doi: 10.1016/S2213-8587(17)30168-7.

DIABETES INFORMATION

1. American Diabetes Association: Provides comprehensive information on diabetes management, research, and advocacy.
    https://www.diabetes.org

2. National Institute of Diabetes and Digestive and Kidney Diseases (NIDDK): Offers detailed information on diabetes research and resources.
    https://www.niddk.nih.gov

3. Centers for Disease Control and Prevention (CDC) - Diabetes: Features statistics, prevention tips, and management strategies.
    https://www.cdc.gov/diabetes

4. Mayo Clinic - Diabetes: Provides medical information and patient resources on diabetes symptoms, diagnosis, and treatment.
    www.mayoclinic.org https://www.mayoclinic.org/diseases-conditions/diabetes

5. WebMD Diabetes Center: Offers articles, tools, and resources for diabetes management and health.
https://www.webmd.com/diabetes

6. Diabetes UK: A leading UK charity providing information, support, and research updates on diabetes.
https://www.diabetes.org.uk

7. Juvenile Diabetes Research Foundation (JDRF): Focuses on type 1 diabetes research, advocacy, and community support.
https://www.jdrf.org

8. National Diabetes Education Program (NDEP): A partnership program that provides educational resources for diabetes prevention and control.
https://www.ndep.nih.gov

9. Beyond Type 1: An online community offering support, resources, and advocacy for individuals with type 1 diabetes.
https://www.beyondtype1.org

10. Diabetes Daily: A community and resource site for diabetes news, recipes, and forums.
https://www.diabetesdaily.com

11. International Diabetes Federation (IDF): Provides global diabetes statistics, resources, and advocacy efforts.
https://www.idf.org

12. T1International: An organization advocating for access to insulin and diabetes supplies globally.
   https://www.t1international.com

13. Children with Diabetes: A site dedicated to families and children living with diabetes, offering support and resources.
   https://www.childrenwithdiabetes.com

14. Diabetes.co.uk: A UK-based site with information, community forums, and resources on diabetes management.
   https://www.diabetes.co.uk

15. My Diabetes My Way: An interactive website to help people manage their diabetes with tools, resources, and personal health records.
   https://www.mydiabetesmyway.scot.nhs.uk

16. DiaTribe: A site providing information on diabetes research, treatments, and patient perspectives.
   https://www.diatribe.org

17. GlucoseZone: A platform offering fitness programs and guidance tailored for people with diabetes.
   https://www.glucosezone.com

18. College Diabetes Network: A resource for college students with diabetes, offering support and advocacy.
   https://www.collegediabetesnetwork.org

19. Insulin Nation: Provides news and information about insulin, diabetes technology, and research.
https://www.insulinnation.com

20. DiabetesStrong: A website focused on fitness and nutrition for people with diabetes, offering workout plans and healthy recipes.
https://www.diabetesstrong.com

These websites offer a wealth of information and support for managing diabetes, from medical advice and research updates to community forums and personal stories.

GLOSSARY

A1C (HbA1c): A test that measures the average blood glucose levels over the past 2-3 months. It indicates how well diabetes is being managed.

Adrenaline: A hormone released during stress or high-intensity exercise, which can increase blood glucose levels.

Autoimmune Disease: A condition in which the immune system attacks the body's own cells, such as the insulin-producing cells in type 1 diabetes.

Basal Insulin: Long-acting insulin that helps maintain blood glucose levels in the absence of meals.

Beta Cells: Cells in the pancreas that produce insulin.

Blood Glucose: The concentration of glucose in the blood, measured in milligrams per deciliter (mg/dL) or millimoles per liter (mmoL/L).

Body Cell Mass (BCM) Body Cell Mass is the living, protein-based, metabolically active tissue in the body, where more over than 90% of the metabolic processes are taking place.

Body Mass Index (BMI) Body Mass Index (BMI) is a simple index of weight-for-height commonly used to classify overweight and obesity in adults. It is computed as weight in kilograms divided by height in meters squared (kg/m2). Ranges from 18.5 to 25 are considered normal, values below 18.5 may indicate malnutrition, values higher than 25 to 30 are defining overweight. Obesity being defined when BMI is 30 or more.

Bolus Insulin: Short-acting insulin taken before meals to manage blood glucose spikes.

Carbohydrate Counting: A method of managing blood glucose levels by tracking the number of carbohydrates consumed in each meal.

Carbohydrates (CHO): A major macronutrient found in foods, which are broken down into glucose and affect blood sugar levels.

Celiac Disease: An autoimmune disorder often associated with type 1 diabetes, where the ingestion of gluten leads to damage in the small intestine.

CGM (Continuous Glucose Monitor): A device that continuously tracks blood glucose levels throughout the day and night.

C-Peptide Test: A test that measures the level of C-peptide in the blood, which can indicate how much insulin the body is producing.

Diabetes Distress: Emotional burden and stress related to managing diabetes.

Diabetic Ketoacidosis (DKA): A serious condition caused by high blood glucose levels and a lack of insulin, leading to the production of ketones and acidosis.

Dawn Phenomenon: An early morning rise in blood glucose levels due to hormonal changes.

Endocrinologist: A doctor who specializes in hormone-related conditions, including diabetes.

Exogenous Insulin: Insulin administered from outside the body.

Extra Cellular Water (ECW) Extra Cellular Water represents the fluids outside the cells. ECW is located mostly in between the cells (interstitial), the blood and lymphatic system.

Fat Mass (FM) The Fat Mass is a compound comprised of glycerol – a substance formed in fatty acids – and fatty acids which is required as a concentrated energy source for our muscles. Fat is a storage compartment for the body's extra calories and it fills fatty cells (adipose tissue) that help insulating the body and protect body organs from trauma.

Fat Free Mass (FFM) Or lean mass is defined as Body weight kg – Fat mass kg. Fat-free mass is the combined mass of the body of everything that is not fat (e.g. muscles, bones, skin and organs)

Fat Oxidation: The process of breaking down fat molecules to produce energy, important in endurance sports.

Fasting Blood Glucose: Blood glucose levels measured after an overnight fast.

Fiasp: A brand of rapid-acting insulin.

Gluconeogenesis: The production of glucose from non-carbohydrate sources, such as amino acids.

Glucagon: A hormone that raises blood glucose levels, used to treat severe hypoglycemia.

Glycemic Control: The management of blood glucose levels within a target range.

Glycemic Index (GI): A measure of how quickly carbohydrates in food raise blood glucose levels.

Glycemic Load (GL): A measure that takes into account both the quality (GI) and quantity of carbohydrates in food.

HbA1c: See A1C.

Hyperglycemia: Higher than normal blood glucose levels, typically above 180 mg/dL.

Hyperinsulinemia: Higher than normal levels of insulin in the blood, often associated with insulin resistance.

Hypoglycemia: Lower than normal blood glucose levels, typically below 70 mg/dL.

Hypoglycemia Unawareness: A condition where a person with diabetes does not feel the usual symptoms of low blood glucose.

Insulin: A hormone that helps cells absorb glucose from the bloodstream.

Insulin Pump: A device that delivers a continuous supply of insulin through a catheter placed under the skin.

Insulin Resistance: A condition where cells do not respond properly to insulin, leading to high blood glucose levels.

Insulin Sensitivity: The degree to which cells respond to insulin, allowing glucose to enter the cells.

Ketoacidosis: See Diabetic Ketoacidosis.

Ketones: Chemicals produced when the body breaks down fat for energy, which can accumulate to dangerous levels in the blood and urine if insulin is insufficient.

Lipohypertrophy: Thickened skin at insulin injection sites caused by repeated injections.

Low-Carb Diet: A diet that restricts carbohydrate intake, typically to less than 130 grams per day.

Macronutrients: The main nutrients in food, including carbohydrates, proteins, and fats.

Marathon: A long-distance running race of 42.195 kilometers (26.2 miles).

Menstrual Cycle: The monthly cycle of changes in the ovaries and the lining of the uterus, which can affect blood glucose levels.

Microalbuminuria: The presence of a small amount of albumin in the urine, an early sign of kidney disease.

Neuropathy: Nerve damage caused by chronic high blood glucose levels.

Nephropathy: Kidney damage caused by chronic high blood glucose levels.

Olympic Triathlon: A triathlon race consisting of a 1.5 km swim, 40 km bike ride, and a 10 km run.

Pancreas: An organ that produces insulin and other important enzymes and hormones.

Phase angle (PhA) Phase Angle represents a mathematical relationship between resistance and reactance. Lower phase angles have been related to increased morbidity and mortality. Target for men is > 6 and women > 5.

Postprandial: Referring to the period after a meal.

Pre-prandial: Referring to the period before a meal.

Protein: A macronutrient essential for growth and repair, important for maintaining muscle mass and overall health.

Retinopathy: Damage to the retina caused by chronic high blood glucose levels.

Self-Monitoring of Blood Glucose (SMBG): Regularly checking blood glucose levels using a glucometer.

Somogyi Effect: A rebound effect where low blood glucose levels during the night cause high blood glucose levels in the morning.

Sprint Triathlon: A short-distance triathlon consisting of a 750 m swim, 20 km bike ride, and a 5 km run.

Stress Hormones: Hormones such as cortisol and adrenaline that are released in response to stress and can affect blood glucose levels.

Total Body Water (TBW) Body Water is expressed as a percentage of weight and includes water that is inside (intracellular) and outside the cells (extracellular). TBW varies depending upon age and gender, it increases with increased muscle mass.

Tresiba: A brand of long-acting insulin.

Type 1 Diabetes: An autoimmune condition where the body attacks and destroys insulin-producing cells in the pancreas.

Type 2 Diabetes: A metabolic disorder characterized by insulin resistance and reduced insulin production.

UKPDS: The United Kingdom Prospective Diabetes Study, a major clinical study that provided important data on the management of type 2 diabetes.

VO2 Max: The maximom rate of oxygen consumption measured during incremental exercise; an indicator of cardiovascular fitness and aerobic endurance.

Zone Training: A method of training that involves exercising at different intensity levels, or "zones," to improve overall fitness and performance.

Zinc: A mineral that plays a role in insulin storage and secretion; important for overall health and immune function.

Zone 1 (Z1): The lowest heart rate zone, typically used for recovery and light aerobic exercise.

Zone 2 (Z2): A moderate heart rate zone that promotes fat oxidation and aerobic endurance.

Zone 3 (Z3): A higher heart rate zone used for improving aerobic capacity and endurance.

Zone 4 (Z4): A high-intensity heart rate zone aimed at improving anaerobic capacity and lactate threshold.

Zone 5 (Z5): The highest heart rate zone, used for short bursts of maximom effort to increase power and speed.

Zigzag Dieting: A nutritional strategy that involves varying caloric intake on different days to prevent metabolic adaptation and promote weight loss or muscle gain.

Zeaxanthin: A carotenoid alcohol found in the retina, important for eye health and potentially protective against diabetic retinopathy.

Zoster Vaccine: A vaccine to prevent shingles, recommended for older adults and individuals with chronic conditions like diabetes, as they are at higher risk for complications.

Zinc Transporter 8 (ZnT8): A protein associated with the regulation of insulin in the pancreas; autoantibodies to ZnT8 are often found in individuals with type 1 diabetes.

Zero-Carb Diet: An extreme form of low-carb diet where all carbohydrates are eliminated; not generally recommended for diabetes management due to nutritional deficiencies and health risks.

Zeta Potential: A scientific term referring to the electric potential in the interfacial double layer of a particle; in medical research, it's sometimes related to drug delivery systems and nanoparticle behavior.

Zenith: The highest point reached by a celestial body; metaphorically used to describe peak performance or health status in athletes or individuals with chronic conditions.

Zoonosis: An infectious disease that can be transmitted from animals to humans; important in the context of diabetes as some zoonotic infections can complicate diabetes management.

Zymogen: An inactive enzyme precursor that requires a biochemical change to become active; relevant in the study of digestive enzymes and insulin production.

9 788889 292223